Emotional Intelligence in Health and Social Care

a guide for improving human relationships

Edited by

John Hurley

Senior Lecturer, Nursing, Southern Cross University, Australia

Paul Linsley

Senior Lecturer, University of Lincoln, UK

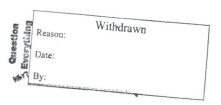
Radcliffe Publishing
London • New York

Radcliffe Publishing Ltd
33-41 Dallington Street
London
EC1V 0BB
United Kingdom

www.radcliffepublishing.com

British Library Cataloguing in Publication Data

A catalogue record for this book is available from the British Library.

ISBN-13: 978 184619 540 2

The paper used for the text pages of this book is FSC® certified. The FSC® (the Forest Stewardship Council®) is an international network to promote responsible management of the world's forests.

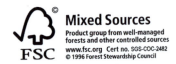

Mixed Sources
Product group from well-managed forests and other controlled sources
www.fsc.org Cert no. SGS-COC-2482
© 1996 Forest Stewardship Council

Typeset by KnowledgeWorks Global Ltd, Chennai, India
Cover designed by Cox Design Ltd, Witney, Oxon, UK
Printed and bound by TJI Digital, Padstow, Cornwall, UK

Contents

Foreword

When people are seriously ill, distressed, or otherwise experiencing problems in their lives, they need help. The kind of help they need may not be clear but they need someone to deliver it; someone who is 'useful', not simply 'well-intentioned'. When gripped by a serious illness, or trapped by apparently insurmountable problems, people have little interest in the helper's qualifications or professional titles. They need something more fundamental than a badge of professional esteem. They want to know: 'what can you do for me?' When people are in pain, upset, or feel their lives have spun out of control, something deeply human is going on. More accurately, such events remind us of our animal natures. When trapped, in pain or otherwise threatened, animals behave in much the same way as humans. Responding to a wounded, fearful animal – of any species – requires much the same response as when a person is hurt, upset or terrified. So what, exactly, is needed, to be helpful?

The simplicity of the answer belies the complexity of its practice. Any hurt, wounded, distressed, frustrated or disconcerted person (or animal) needs to be *understood*. This is not a big ask but, paradoxically, in professional settings there is no bigger challenge. The traditional professional ethic is 'first, do no harm'. A more fundamental ethic might be: 'first, seek understanding; only then can you make yourself understood'.

By contrast, professional helpers from all disciplines tend, traditionally, to 'know' their patients, clients, upset or troubled people, as *things* somehow separate from them. They are studied through the various lenses of biology, psychology, sociology and other 'ologies' which lose the individual distressed, hurting person in the process. We try to know 'about' the physiological or psychological roots of pain, or the sociological ramifications of panic, expecting that we can apply this knowledge to make a difference. In practice, professionals often focus on trying to make themselves understood – explaining the problem, emphasising what needs to be done and why – *before* they make any attempt to understand what is happening for the person. Scientific and other forms of professional knowledge may provide useful 'tools' but first we need to understand what is needed. Only then can decisions be made – hopefully, conjointly with the person – as to what 'tools' might be appropriate and when.

This is all about human relationships – the relations we have with others and the relations we have with ourselves: nothing more; nothing less. We cannot begin to make contact with a frightened, wounded person (or animal) without first *understanding* what is happening. We *recognise* this because we see, hear and *feel* things that remind us of our own understandings of fear, pain etc. When our own feelings of hurt or fear are 'stirred up' by our contact with a distressed person, we need to be able to manage our own distress, if we are to be of any use to the other person. Knowing ourselves and being able to deal with our own emotions is a prerequisite for knowing and helping others.

This book is about 'emotional intelligence', which is one of the names for the abstract, invisible processes that people appear to use in their relationships with themselves, and as part of their relating, effectively, meaningfully or helpfully with others. As the various authors discuss, there is much debate over the definition of emotional intelligence, or even its legitimacy as a concept, but it seems clear that without it – whatever 'it' is – most areas of human endeavour would not be possible. As Darwin first speculated in his early work, the emotions play a vital role in our survival and also in learning how to adapt to changing circumstances. Again, this is as true for animals in the wild as for humans in contemporary society.

When I began my professional training over 40 years ago the curriculum paid no attention to the 'stuff' of the 'emotions'. Indeed, when someone was described as 'emotional', invariably this meant that they were in some dysfunctional state. Cold, calculating reason was needed to provide a counterbalance. So we genuflected before the altar of reason, buried our noses in books, trying to digest the 'facts' about the world and its inhabitants. However, when faced with the confusion of real people, and the uncertainty of decision making, I – like everyone else – had to draw on my emotions; *feeling* my way towards a different kind of knowledge. Forty years ago I would have welcomed a book like this with open arms. It might have helped me understand better my 'emotional intelligence'. It might even have helped me come to a different understanding of what I needed to do to help myself to coexist with, work alongside and help others.

Phil Barker
Psychotherapist in Private Practice
Honorary Professor
University of Dundee, Scotland

Preface

Emotional Intelligence in Health and Social Care: a guide for improving human relationships is an essential resource for practitioners, educationalists and clinical teachers engaged in providing care for others. Readers of this book will gain a theoretical understanding of emotional intelligence (EI) and its practical application to medicine, nursing and social work, as well as allied health and clinical leadership roles. Through gaining these understandings it is hoped that students and practitioners will have a significantly expanded range of therapeutic responses to care for others, whilst simultaneously developing themselves.

The challenges of achieving meaningful therapeutic relations are becoming more complex with shorter and more focused interventions being the increasing norm within health and social care environments. Additionally, these care interventions are becoming more reliant on mechanised, pharmaceutical and other related products as our knowledge of effective treatments expands. This combination of short-term relating and product-focused interventions creates the very real potential for the personal dimensions of care to be diminished for both the givers and recipients of care. This book offers the knowledge and behaviours to respond to these contemporary, challenging contexts of care delivery. The divergent authors of the chapters within this book are all highly experienced practitioners who apply the *inter*personal and *intra*personal capabilities of emotional intelligence to providing evidenced based and yet personalised interventions. Their knowledge and understandings will empower the reader to be more enabled in achieving these outcomes. While emphasising caring for others, this book also places great importance on the practitioner caring for and developing him or herself.

Contemporary care environments place high demands upon students and practitioners of all disciplines. The authors of this book want practitioners to do more than simply survive these environments, they want practitioners to thrive and feel enabled to lead themselves and others. The individual and collaborative reflective exercises within this book offer ways to achieve these ends. The reflective exercises and activities will also guide the reader toward achieving a better understanding of how to work effectively with the diversity of other professionals who make up multidisciplinary care teams.

Education for practitioners is increasingly cluttered with keeping abreast of evidenced-based developments, mandatory training requirements and knowledge pertaining to the increasing complexities and expansion of professional roles. This book offers a balanced approach to the interpersonal and intrapersonal dimensions of effectively caring for others.

To help the reader make the most of the text, reflective exercises are interspersed within each of the chapters. As well as adding interest to the text they encourage readers to think about the issue under debate and integrate the material with their own understanding of clinical practice and healthcare.

We hope that you enjoy the book.

John Hurley and Paul Linsley

About the editors

John Hurley

Dr John Hurley is a qualified nurse, mental health nurse and psychotherapist, and is currently working as a Senior Lecturer at Southern Cross University in Coffs Harbour, Australia. John has had a long clinical career working and leading services within challenging fields of health and with people experiencing great distress. He now lectures and researches on communication, mental health and leadership.

Paul Linsley

Paul Linsley began his nursing career as a general nurse working within acute medicine. Following conversion to mental health nursing he gained valuable experience in a variety of clinical settings. Paul is registered as a Clinical Specialist in Acute Psychiatry and is trained in cognitive behavioural therapy; he is also a Lead Trainer in Conflict Resolution and Management. As a Senior Lecturer for the University of Lincoln he teaches on a number of courses, single and joint-honours undergraduate programmes, research masters programmes and pre- and post-registration nurse training programmes.

About the contributors

Derek Barron

Since October 2007, Derek has been the Associate Nurse Director of Mental Health Services in NHS Ayrshire and Arran. He has spent significant time on staff development, evidencing an underlying belief that learning organisations are made up of learning people. In addition to his Associate Nurse Director role, Derek was Chair of the Mental Health Nursing Forum Scotland in 2009; this forum has representatives from each of the Scottish NHS Boards and also the NHS Education Scotland, NHS Quality Improvement Scotland, Mental Welfare Commission, Care Commission and Higher Education Institutes. Derek is on the Editorial Board of the *British Journal of Wellbeing*.

Valeria Carroll

Valeria Carroll is a Senior Lecturer in Social Care (Child Studies) and BSc Psychology with Child Studies pathway co-ordinator with the University of Lincoln. Dr Carroll studied and received her BSc (psychologist-pedagogue), MSc (developmental psychology) and PhD (individual differences) degrees in Moscow before making her way from to the UK from Russia. Dr Carroll began her career as an organisational psychologist and then went on to be an educational psychologist before joining the health education sector. Her research interests are devoted to principles of assessment and individual differences.

Kim Foster

Kim has been a mental health nurse for over 25 years and is currently Associate Professor of Mental Health Nursing at Sydney Nursing School, University of Sydney. As a mental health nurse Kim has had a longstanding interest in the use of emotional intelligence in practice, and she teaches interpersonal nursing theory and skills to pre- and post-registration nurses. Her research areas include resilience in children and families where parents have mental illness; emotional intelligence in healthcare professionals; and the interface between physical and mental health.

Nigel Horner

Nigel has been engaged in social work education since 1995. He joined the University of Lincoln from Nottingham Trent University in 2007. Nigel is the author of *What is Social Work?* (2006) and *Social Work in Education and Children's Services* (2006), and is currently co-editing a book on social work values.

Natalie Liddle

Natalie Liddle is currently studying towards her BSc Honors in adult nursing at the University of Lincoln. She is a passionate individual and has a great enthusiasm for nursing. Natalie has achieved great success in a number of research projects in her faculty of health, life and social sciences and is currently working on a number of publishing projects. Natalie plays an active role in student life as president of the newly formed Nursing Society, for which she actively represents students across her faculty and university. She has recently received recognition for her efforts while at the university and has been awarded the prestigious John Jenkins Award, given to students that show outstanding commitment to both the student union and the university. Natalie currently holds positions within organisations nationally. She has a keen interest in emotional intelligence within nursing and hopes to progress into the field of palliative care.

Heather McKenzie

Heather McKenzie is a Senior Lecturer and Associate Dean (Learning & Teaching) at Sydney Nursing School, University of Sydney. Her research interests include cancer survivorship and cancer care, social theory, the interface between acute and community services, and pre-registration nursing education. Heather currently leads a team of researchers seeking to identify and address unmet needs of chemotherapy outpatients. Heather teaches in the social sciences stream of the pre-registration Master of Nursing course at Sydney Nursing School and is also involved in research into a range of different aspects of nursing student experiences.

Bob Rankin

Dr Bob Rankin is a Senior Lecturer in Undergraduate and Postgraduate Mental Health Nursing at the University of Dundee. His research interests include emotional intelligence and its relationship with academic attainment, practice performance and attrition in nurse education. Bob entered nurse education in the late 1980s following five years as a charge nurse in a mental health day hospital for people under the age of 65. He is a member of the Mental Health Nursing Forum (Scotland) and Mental Health Nursing Academics UK.

Charlie Stansfield

Charlie Stansfield is a writer and social worker who grew up in Newcastle upon Tyne and studied in Leeds. She worked in the community sector until the late 1980s, when Margret Thatcher caused her to flee to Auckland, New Zealand. Charlie has postgraduate qualifications in family therapy, narrative therapy and management in the not-for-profit sector. She currently lives and works in Sydney as a grief counsellor and freelance journalist.

List of figures

List of tables

List of boxes

Dedication

John and I would like to dedicate this book to my son, Andrew James Linsley, who tragically died in an accident on New Year's Day this year, aged 20.

The following is a poem written by Amy, one of Andrew's friends, on hearing the news of his death. It demonstrates the power of emotional expression and provides a fitting tribute to a lost loved one.

The Tribute Ale

The rhythmic droning consumed us to a pleasant emptiness,
Where Andrew had not died,
And our lives were not frozen in pain.
We all huddled together each in our stages of grief and were as one
Each friend an extension of another's essence
The loss of a friend to a vague emptiness and confusion
Will force moments to last for hours
This was not supposed to have happened.
The strange parallel world where we are no longer amongst the living.
As I watched the fires go out in the sky, I saw towers of men crumble into the stairs
You have not died,
You are far too alive,
You will always live,
I have died.

CHAPTER 1

Introducing emotional intelligence

John Hurley

Whether you are newly entering a health or social care profession, or are perhaps an experienced practitioner, being good at what you do will require more than having academic knowledge about your field of work. You will frequently be called upon to simultaneously foster positive patient experiences of receiving high quality care, while also coping with the multiple stressors, practical dilemmas and emotional demands that are part and parcel of helping others (Holmes 2006).

Modern expectations of health or social care practitioners are that you have the capacity to develop the skills, intrapersonal capabilities and interpersonal capabilities to respond to such demands. These skills and capabilities can be organised into any number of frameworks such as 'specialist capabilities'; a hierarchal model such as 'beginner and 'advanced' capabilities', or as outlined in this book: as skills and capabilities that are about being emotionally intelligent. Through exploring emotionally intelligent capabilities we hope to make you more aware of effective ways to respond to the challenges on personal and professional levels.

INTELLIGENCE

Before exploring emotional intelligence (EI) let us take a step back to consider and clarify what is meant by the term 'intelligence'. We are going to briefly explore some of the different ways to understand what it means to be 'intelligent'. Before we do this, however, try out the social-based activity below to gain an insight into what others in your profession and personal life believe intelligence to be.

Box 1.1   Social-based activity

Over the next week ask 10 people what they think intelligence is. Ensure you get them to give you at least three characteristics of their understanding of intelligence.

If you have opportunity, make half of these people from your chosen profession, and ask them what an 'intelligent physiotherapist' or an 'intelligent social worker' is.

Compare findings with your peers or in class and build a picture of common understandings toward 'intelligence'.

Traditional understanding of intelligence

Traditional understandings of the term 'intelligence' are that it refers to the academically grounded ability measured through a traditional IQ test. This understanding of intelligence focuses upon individuals' abilities to solve problems, apply reason and to think in abstract terms. IQ tests, of which the Wechsler Adult Intelligence Scale III is perhaps one of the best known, have been in place for nearly 100 years, and can be best understood as comprising of four areas which together make up intelligence:
1   verbal comprehension
2   perceptual organisation
3   processing speed
4   working memory (Deary 2001).

Box 1.2 Web-based activity

Using academic, professional and even public data base sources, explore the term 'intelligence testing'.

Testing is a vital area to explore, as these tests reflect the capabilities that are agreed upon to represent what intelligence is (otherwise the test would be invalid).

Identify, list and reflect upon the testing content you find as part of your search.

A key reflective question is: does human functioning extend beyond the abilities measured by these tests?

Arguably many of you may have came to the conclusion that human functioning is more than what can be measured by tests such as the Wechsler Adult Intelligence Scale III. However, can we label these additional abilities as 'intelligence' or are they associated with other areas of human functioning?

Multiple intelligences

The idea of multiple intelligences is that there are intelligences beyond the traditional idea of intelligence as measured by standard psychometric testing. Social and interpersonal intelligence was forwarded by Hunt (1928) and Strang (1930), each highlighting abilities in dealing with other people. Hence the application of the term 'intelligence' to abilities outside of IQ alone; this thinking can also be seen as having a long tradition and was expanded upon by Sternberg (1997), who recognised key differences between academic problem-solving capability (intelligence) and real-world problem-solving (also called intelligence). Sternberg (1997) broke down what different challenges academic and real world problems posed:

Academic problems are seen as:

1 being set by others
2 being well-defined
3 being complete with information
4 having only one correct answer and one means to achieve that answer
5 having little intrinsic interest.

Alternatively, practical or 'real world' problems are seen as:

1 being unformulated
2 lacking complete information
3 being poorly defined
4 having multiple correct answers, but each solution having both liabilities and advantages
5 being of personal interest (Sternberg and Grigorenko 2000, pp. 215–43).

Both of these lists hold their own challenges to the individuals' ability and are prefaced by Sternberg (1997) as requiring 'practical intelligence' to alter the immediate environment so as to solve real-world problems. This practical intelligence is broken down by Sternberg and Grigorenko (2000) as:

1 recognising and defining problems
2 allocating resources to address the problem
3 mentally representing the problem
4 formulating ways to solve problems
5 evaluating the efficacy of problem-solving strategies.

Practical intelligence is focused toward the immediate circumstances facing the individual, and as such there is an enormous variety of ways in which individuals may well employ practical intelligence strategies. Keep this list in mind when next in practise and observe fellow professionals you judge as being highly capable to see if they display this practical intelligence.

While one might presume that greater practical experience will automatically lead to greater practical intelligence and hence problem-solving ability, this is not always the case. Within practice environments there will be complexity, unpredictability and hence uncertainty (Sorrentino *et al.* 2008). While you may be confronted with similar clinical problems, the context of that presentation will alter every time, possibly requiring you to use different strategies.

Social intelligence

The theory of social or multiple intelligences was developed in 1983 by Dr Howard Gardner, professor of education at Harvard University. It suggests that the traditional notion of intelligence, based on IQ testing, is far too limited. Instead, Gardner proposes eight different intelligences to account for a broader range of human potential. These intelligences are:

1   linguistic intelligence (words and language)
2   logical-mathematical intelligence (logic and numbers)
3   spatial intelligence (images and space)
4   bodily kinaesthetic intelligence (body movement control)
5   musical intelligence (music, sound, rhythm)
6   interpersonal intelligence (other people's feelings)
7   intrapersonal intelligence (self-awareness)
8   naturalist intelligence (natural environment).

The central tenant of social intelligence is that humans are reflective, cognisant beings who attempt to make sense of and meet their needs within a social-based reality (Cantor and Kihlstrom 1987). Gardner's view is that these different types of intelligence work cooperatively and that they are focused upon solving everyday problems. Gardner proposed that multiple intelligences were not limited to his original list, and he has since considered the existence and definitions of other possible intelligences in his later work (1993, 1999). An additional two he has suggested are:

1   religious intelligence ('ultimate issues')
2   moral intelligence (ethics, humanity, value of life).

Not surprisingly, commentators and theorists continually debate and interpret potential additions to the model. Others include the ability to understand and appropriately respond to the feelings, thoughts and behaviours of self and others in interpersonal situations, or as an ability to understand the feelings, thoughts and intentions of others (Marlowe 1986, Silberman 2000).

Box 1.3   Social-based activity

Identify and list the intelligence types within Gardner's framework that you believe yourself to be either strong, or perhaps lacking in. Choose a trusted peer and as a pair evaluate each other's list.

What should emerge for you now is that there are new understandings of what might be constituted as being 'intelligent'.

PERSONALITY OR INTELLIGENCE?

In the previous section we examined the multiplicity of ways of understanding what intelligence is. We also briefly explored how intelligence can be broadly understood as an ability that enables us to meet and effectively respond to the variety of demands arising from our personal needs and professional roles. However, before moving into a more detailed review of EI we need to also briefly explore the construct of personality.

We have identified the ability to understand others and respond to their moods as being 'intelligent', but where does this broad understanding of what intelligence 'is' end and the construct of personality begin? In short, is the person who picks up on the mood of others 'intelligent', or can he alternatively be seen as having a caring 'personality', or perhaps as overlapping between being intelligent and having a caring personality?

Personality can be understood from a variety of perspectives and at its most basic level can be seen as our enduring patterns of behaviour and our personal identity (Butcher 2008). Personality may be seen as behavioural patterns of our thoughts and emotions that remain fairly consistent throughout our life. Note that personality is a cluster of enduring behavioural patterns rather than one-off or isolated behaviours. Hence, personality can be seen as a pervasive behavioural pattern toward ourselves, those around us, and our environment and includes items such as attitudes and perceptions. Whilst far from being an area of universal agreement, the development of personality appears to be a mixture of biological, psychological and sociological influences (Mayer 2005). Of importance to us is that personality is formed early in life and remains very difficult to alter in latter life.

Personality is hence a relatively predictable way in which a person will behave across a variety of circumstances. While personality can be seen by others through what we do (our behaviours), personality is also within our emotions and thoughts as well as being manifest within the way in which we relate to other people; it is that which makes us distinctive. You may also come across the term 'traits' when exploring what personality is. A personality trait can be understood as a singular characteristic that marks you as being different from others, as distinct from personality, which is a cluster of traits. While there are very many individual traits, the well-known example of 'five-factor theory' suggests people have five core traits that make up personality, namely those of:
1   extraversion
2   agreeableness
3   conscientiousness
4   neuroticism
5   openness (Goldberg 1993).

EI is not personality, although the most heated debate surrounding EI is focused on this very issue. Some researchers suggest that many EI measures include measures of personality, while some EI models include personality traits (Conte 2005). However, there remains a clear distinction between personality and EI in terms of its current theoretical modelling (Mayer *et al.* 2008).

Before moving on to explore EI models in more detail, first spend some time to explore the construct of personality. By looking at personality tests you can gain an understanding of what personality is.

Box 1.4 Web-based activity

Look at some online personality tests to gain a sense of what items are considered to be part of 'personality'. This website is one example: www.bbc.co.uk/labuk/experiments/personality

---

EMOTIONAL INTELLIGENCE

Emotional intelligence has been defined as: 'the ability to monitor one's own and other's feelings, to discriminate among them and to use this information to guide one's thinking and actions' (Grewal and Salovey 2005, p. 333). As a result, we make decisions based not only after assessing their outcome, but also on the emotional qualities associated with the decisions or judgements (Grewal and Salovey 2005). This definition of EI explains, in part, the interest and use of EI capabilities across a range of health and social care contexts such as leadership (Akerjordet and Severinsson 2008, Burdett Trust 2009), organisational behaviour (Guleryuz *et al.* 2008), therapeutic relationships (O'Connell 2008), and education (Chabeli 2008, Wilson and Carryer 2008).

However, amongst this blossoming interest in EI there remain genuine tensions as to what precisely is included and excluded from its parameters. We are going to critically explore three major views of EI, the first being EI as an ability model separate from personality by Mayer *et al.* (2008), and then the models of Bar-On (2000) and Goleman (1995), who both offer EI as a fusion of ability and personality trait.

Box 1.5 Reflection activity

There is some worth as you read on in considering and then critically reflecting on how the abilities explained below will help you in your clinical and academic work experiences.

The emotional intelligence model of Mayer *et al.*

Locke (2005) forwards that such is the misuse of the term 'EI' and the palpable over-inclusiveness of abilities attributed to EI that there is no longer validity in its name.

Such views are strongly echoed by Mayer *et al.* (2008), who forward their own 'four-branch model' of EI as being the superior, empirically scientific and conceptually organised approach to EI. In doing so, Mayer *et al.* (2008) continue a longstanding discussion to anchor EI to its original concepts, derived and established through a researched evidence base that show personal and social advantages for people with high emotional clarity (Salovey and Mayer 1990).

Their four-branch model of EI basically consists of a hierarchy of abilities ascending from:

1   the ability to perceive emotions in oneself and others accurately
2   the ability to use emotions to facilitate thinking
3   the ability to understand emotions, emotional language, and the signals conveyed by emotions
4   the ability to manage emotions so as to attain specific goals (Mayer and Salovey 1997).

Within each of these four branches there are subsets of hierarchical abilities that move from the fundamental to the more sophisticated. Central to this model is that EI is an ability that enhances the relationship between emotion and cognition.

Each of the four branches to the model are explained and detailed below:

Stage one of the model focuses upon emotional perception or the picking up on emotions that in turn influence how and what we think. Without this foundational ability to perceive emotions, none of the subsequent steps would be possible.

1   Stage one involves the ability to perceive emotions in one's self and others accurately as:
    • the ability to identify emotion in physical states
    • the ability to identify emotions in other people or items (such as artwork) through mediums of language, sound, and/or behaviour
    • the ability to express emotions accurately and to express needs related to those feelings
    • the ability to discriminate between accurate and inaccurate expressions of feeling.

Stage two of the model then focuses more upon the emotional integration with cognition as the emotions enter active individual awareness. Here, emotions are labeled and influence cognitions either positively or negatively. Perceptions can also be altered.

2   Stage two involves the ability to use emotions to facilitate thinking as follows:
    • emotions prioritise thinking by focusing attention toward important information
    • emotions are sufficiently within the individual's awareness so as to be used in assisting judgment and memory concerning feelings

- emotions influence perspective encouraging consideration of multiple points of view
- emotional states influence specific problem-solving approaches.

Stage three of the model highlights emotional understanding as distinct from merely recognising emotions. Key abilities include truly understanding how emotions influence individuals and individuals within relationships over time.

3   Stage three involves the ability to understand emotions, emotional language, and the signals conveyed by emotions as:
- the ability to differentiate emotions
- the ability to interpret the meanings that emotions convey
- the ability to understand complex feelings that may be multiple and simultaneous
- the ability to recognise possible movement of emotions from one emotional experience to another.

Stage four of the ability model focuses upon the management of the emotion. At this point it is important to note that this framework of understanding emotions is not about the denial and/or avoidance of emotions within personal or professional roles. Rather, it is uncovering how through recognising and understanding the emotions of ourselves and others that we can attain desired outcomes.

4   Stage four involves the ability to manage emotions so as to attain specific goals as:
- the ability to stay open to, yet not be overwhelmed by, emotions
- the ability to engage or detach from emotion depending upon its use
- the ability to monitor emotions in relation to oneself and others
- the ability to manage emotion in oneself and others and flexibly choose a course of action that best fits needs (Mayer and Salovey 1997).

Mayer *et al.* (2008, p. 504) respectively describe other leading figures within the EI debate, such as Bar-On (2000), as including 'unrelated attributes' in his model of EI, and Goleman (1995) as being 'journalistic' (presumably as distinct from scientific) towards EI. Both are mixed approaches that see EI as a fusion of competencies and personality traits, rather than as an ability.

The emotional intelligence model of Bar-On

Bar-On (2000, p. 365) offers EI as a fusion of emotional and social competencies, skills and what Bar-on calls 'facilitators' that all combine to enable intelligent behaviours. Bar-On identifies assertiveness, stress management, self-awareness and flexibility all as being components of EI. Indeed, Bar-On (2000) extends EI into a 15-aspect model arranged in a five-level hierarchical structure:

Level 1   Intrapersonal EI (self-awareness and self-expression)
- self-regard (being aware of, understanding and accepting ourselves)
- emotional self-awareness (being aware of and understanding our emotions)
- assertiveness (expressing our feelings and ourselves non-destructively)
- independence (being self-reliant and free of emotional dependency on others)
- self-actualisation (setting and achieving goals to actualise our potential)

Level 2   Interpersonal EI (social awareness and interaction)
- empathy (being aware of and understanding how others feel)
- social responsibility (identifying with and feeling part of our social groups)
- interpersonal relationship (establishing mutually satisfying relationships)

Level 3   Adaptability EI (change management)
- reality testing (validating our feelings and thinking with external reality)
- flexibility (coping with and adapting to change in our daily life)
- problem-solving (generating effective solutions to problems of an intrapersonal and interpersonal nature)

Level 4   Stress management EI (emotional management and control)
- stress tolerance (effectively and constructively managing our emotions)
- impulse control (effectively and constructively controlling our emotions)

Level 5   General mood EI (self-motivation)
- optimism (having a positive outlook and looking at the brighter side of life)
- happiness (feeling content with ourselves, others and life in general)

(From Bar-On *et al.* Copyright ©2000 John Wiley & Sons Inc. Reproduced with permission of John Wiley & Sons Inc.)

Central to Bar-On's position (2000, p. 373) is that EI is of its very essence the ability to understand, be aware of and also express emotions, and that while very closely related to social intelligence, it is separate from it.

Box 1.6   Reflection activity

Compare and contrast aspects of Bar-on and Mayer *et al.* models and identify areas of possible contrast or crossover. For example, both models have self-awareness at the beginning, suggestive that this is essential to enable the remaining components of the EI capabilities. Conversely, Mayer *et al.* would possibly shun the idea of having a general mood component highlighting happiness and optimism.

The emotional intelligence model of Goleman

The third and final EI model to be explored is that of Daniel Goleman (1995), who arguably moved EI into a wider public awareness with emphasis on organisations, and leadership in particular. His broader interpretations of EI include self-motivation, empathy and relationship skills, as well as impulse control, problem-solving and social responsibility (Goleman 1995, p. 26). The Consortium for Research on Emotional Intelligence in Organisations (1998) and Boyatzis *et al.* (2000) offer a structured framework of EI arising from Goleman's original work.

This framework separates EI capabilities into 4 areas:

1   the capability to *recognise* features of EI within *self*
2   the capability to recognise features of EI constructs within others
3   the capability to *regulate* features of EI constructs within *self*
4   the capability to *regulate* features of EI constructs within *others.*

Expanding upon these key EI capabilities from Goleman's model as detailed by Cherniss *et al.* (1998) demonstrates a notable volume of EI capabilities (*See* Table 1.1 below).

When viewing this quadrant observe how EI capability is initially separated into capabilities focused toward self and others. In turn, this is again separated into EI capabilities to have awareness toward self and others and then separated again into regulating self and others. Table 1.2 offers a more detailed description of the EI capabilities within this model.

What is highlighted by the competencies in the above tables is that the application of EI extends beyond clinical considerations alone and into the dynamic environments where care is delivered. This environment is frequently complex and subject to rapid and at times unpredictable change. Health and social care often struggle to respond quickly to such changes, placing the onus on the staff who work

TABLE 1.1 EI capabilities (adapted from Consortium for Research on Emotional Intelligence in Organisations, 1998)

	Self: personal competence	*Other: social competence*
Recognition	**Self-awareness** • Emotional self-awareness • Accurate self-assessment • Self-confidence	**Social awareness** • Empathy • Service orientation • Organisational awareness
Regulation	**Self-management** • Self-control • Trustworthiness • Conscientiousness • Adaptability • Achievement drive • Initiative	**Relationship management** • Developing others • Influence • Communication • Conflict management • Leadership • Change catalyst • Building bonds • Teamwork • Collaboration

TABLE 1.2 An expanded view of the framework of emotional competencies (adapted from Consortium for Research on Emotional Intelligence in Organisations 1998)

Self: personal competence

Self-awareness
- Emotional self-awareness: know which emotions they are feeling and why; have a guiding awareness of their values and goals
- Accurate self-assessment: show a sense of humour and perspective about themselves; reflective, learning from experience
- Self-confidence: be able to make sound decisions despite uncertainties and pressures; present themselves with self-assurance

Self-management
- Self-control: manage impulsive feelings and distressing emotions; think clearly and stay focused under pressure
- Trustworthiness: build trust through reliability and authenticity; admit one's own mistakes and confront unethical actions in others
- Conscientiousness: meet commitments and keep promises; hold self accountable for meeting his/her objectives
- Adaptability: smoothly handle shifting priorities and rapid change; adapt responses and tactics to fit fluid circumstances
- Achievement drive: results-oriented with a high drive; set challenging goals and take calculated risks
- Initiative: pursue goals beyond what's required or expected; mobilise others through unusual, enterprising efforts

Other: social competence

Social awareness
- Empathy: show sensitivity and understand others' perspectives; help out based on understanding other people's needs and feelings
- Service orientation: gladly offer appropriate assistance; grasp a customer's perspective, act as a trusted advisor
- Leverage diversity: respect and relate well to people from varied backgrounds; understand diverse worldviews

Relationship management
- Develop others: identify people's needs for development; mentor and offer assignments that challenge and grow a person's skill
- Influence: use complex strategies to build consensus and support; orchestrate dramatic events to make a point effectively
- Communication: listen well, seek mutual understanding; foster open communication and stay receptive to bad news as well as good
- Conflict management: handle difficult people and tense situations with diplomacy and tact; spot potential conflict and deescalate
- Leadership: guide the performance of others while holding them accountable; lead by example
- Change catalyst: recognise the need for change and remove barriers; challenge the status quo to acknowledge the need for change

(Continued)

TABLE 1.2 An expanded view of the framework of emotional competencies (adapted from Consortium for Research on Emotional Intelligence in Organisations 1998) (Continued)

Self: personal competence

- Building bonds: cultivate and maintain extensive informal networks; seek out relationships that are mutually beneficial
- Teamwork: model team qualities like respect, helpfulness and cooperation; draw all members into active and enthusiastic participation
- Collaboration: balance a focus on task with attention to relationships; collaborate by sharing plans, information and resources

within them to adjust (Hurley and Linsley 2007, Limerick *et al.* 2002, p. 83). It is from within this challenging environment that health and social care practitioners must have the intrapersonal and interpersonal capabilities to respond to their clients' needs, as well as their own needs.

Box 1.7 Social activity

At this point there is some worth in stopping to apply how the abilities described in this EI model have pertained to your own practice-based experiences, and experiences within other social roles you have. Review the list of capabilities in this EI model with a trusted peer and how you have used these capabilities (or not).

* Having an understanding of EI now means that you can begin to develop aspects of your own EI. When doing the social and reflective activities in these chapters, identify any of your own emotions that will emerge. For example, when asked to reveal aspects of yourself with a trusted peer, what did you feel: did you choose that peer or did he choose you, and what might that be about? Did your feelings impact on your actions such as possibly feeling fearful of sharing and hence not participating?

Emotional intelligence measures

Some of you may be wondering how to resolve the differences between the models of EI that we have explored, while perhaps others may be intrigued to know what level of EI you may have. Both these issues can be addressed through a very brief look at the measurement of EI. Within this consideration is the question of whether what is being measured is actually something new, i.e. EI, or is it measuring a repackaging of personality traits already effectively measured by psychometric tests that we simply label as EI?

Mayer *et al.* (2000, 2004) identify EI as ability and view other competence EI models that include leadership or assertiveness as failing in content validity with their measures. In other words, Mayer *et al.* (2000, 2004) claim they are measuring EI while others are simply measuring personality traits. They offer empirical support for their EI model through their 'Mayer, Salovey, Caruso Emotional Intelligence Test' (MSCEIT). The MSCEIT reflects the working theory that EI is a specific ability to process the information pertaining to emotional perception, emotional facilitation of thought, emotional understanding and finally, emotional management. As such the MSCEIT is a performance measure, as it directly connects intelligence to ability. In common with other ability measures it has a higher correlation to cognitive ability than the mixed EI models such as Bar-On (2000) and Goleman (1995) (Van Rooy *et al.* 2005).

By contrast, Bar-On's self-report measure, the 133-itemed Emotional Quotient Inventory (EQ-i) – based upon a Likert Scale – culminates in a global EI score, as well as individual scores for each composite item that constitutes Bar-On's model of EI. This self reporting tool has internal validity indicators and has been normed across international populations (Bar-on 2000). The EQ-360, a multi-rater tool, has also been developed.

Boyatzis *et al.* (2000) outline the Emotional Competence Inventory (ECI), a measurement tool reflecting Goleman's model of EI (1995). As with the other EI approaches, the measurement tool was worked outwards from the model, strengthening the validity of outcomes. The ECI 2.0, also based on Goleman's model, is a multi-rater, 360-degree tool designed to assess the emotional and social competencies of individuals in organisations.

The ECI, as with all the other mixed measurement tools, appear to show that there is both a crossover between existing understandings and measures of personality and that of EI; these tools also find areas distinctive to EI (Byrne *et al.* 2007). Additionally, mixed measurement tools show a greater correlation with personality and a lower correlation with cognitive capability than ability or performance tools (Van Rooy *et al.* 2005).

While the view of EI is partially opaque, there arguably exists enough clarity and agreement upon EI capabilities to proceed with a cautious exploration of EI in relation to the roles of practitioners. Before commencing this exploration one final question needs to be addressed; that of 'Can EI capabilities be improved?'

Education and training for emotional intelligence

Having offered both an understanding of EI and some initial links between EI and professional roles it is important that we consider if your EI capabilities can be altered through education and/or training.

Cherniss *et al.* (1998) sought responses to this question through a robust exploration of literature. As a result of this reviewing it emerged that the process of developing EI requires motivation to change, and that the change sought is the change within and about oneself, and oneself in relation to others. Successful enhancement of EI capability also requires educational approaches that are individually packaged and self-directed. Individual learning styles need to be catered for and the learner positioned to be in charge of the program. Other key areas of educating for improved EI include:

- setting specific behavioural goals that are clear and challenging
- practising the behavioural goals over a period of months both at work and in life utilising naturally occurring opportunities
- utilising experiential methods that are active and concrete
- genuine modelling from high-status persons within on-the-job contexts
- enhancing self-awareness that is central to developing EI, which is the cornerstone of emotional and social competence
- generating an organisational culture that is safe for experimentation with the new behaviours (Boyatzis 2002, Cherniss *et al.* 1998).

CHAPTER SUMMARY

This chapter has hopefully triggered some thinking about the importance of health and social care practitioners having a range of inter- and intrapersonal capabilities to adequately fulfil their professional roles. The chapter has also introduced you to the idea that there are multiple ways of understanding what intelligence is, and that this multiple understanding includes EI.

EI can be understood as being either separate from or partially overlapping with the construct of personality depending upon the EI model. Regardless of the EI model adopted, this chapter has pinpointed specific EI capabilities that are essential to successfully engage in caring for others, and that it appears to be very possible to become better at being emotionally intelligent when motivated to do so and supported by your environment.

The subsequent chapters of this book now seek to not only build on your motivation to improve your EI capabilities, but to also offer ways to do so.

REFERENCES

Akerjordet K, Severinsson E. Emotionally intelligent nurse leadership: a literature review study. *J Nurs Manag.* 2008; **16**(5): 565–77.

Bar-On R, editor. *The Handbook of Emotional Intelligence: the theory and practice of development, evaluation, education and implementation – at home, school and the workplace.* San Francisco, CA: Jossey-Bass; 2000.

Boyatzis R, Goleman D, Rhee K. Clustering competence in emotional intelligence: insights from the emotional competence inventory. In: Bar-On, op. cit. pp. 343–62.

Burdett Trust. *The Nurse Executives' Handbook: leading the business of caring from ward to board.* London: The King's Fund; 2009.

Butcher J. *Personality Assessment in Treatment Planning*. Oxford: Oxford University Press; 2008.

Byrne J, Dominick P, Smither J, *et al*. Examination of the discriminate, convergent, and criterion-related validity of self-ratings on the Emotional Competence Inventory. *International Journal of Selection and Assessment*. 2007; **15**(3): 341–53.

Cantor N, Kihlstrom J. *Personality and Social Intelligence*. Englewood Cliffs, NJ: Eribaum; 1987.

Chabeli M. Humor: a pedagogical tool to promote learning. *Curationis*. 2008; **31**(3): 51–9.

Cherniss C, Goleman D, Emmerling R, *et al*. (1998). *Guidelines for Best Practice*. Available at: www.eiconsortium.org/reports/guidelines.html (accessed 20 February 2008).

Consortium for Research on Emotional Intelligence in Organisations. *Emotional Competence Framework*. Available at: www.eiconsortium.org/reports/emotional_competence_framework.html (accessed 26 November 2008).

Conte J. A review and critique of emotional intelligence measures. *J Organ Behav*. 2005; **26**: 433–40.

Deary IJ. Human intelligence differences: a recent history. *Trends Cogn Sci*. 2001; **5**: 127–30.

Gardner H. *Multiple Intelligences: the theory in practice*. New York: Basic Books; 1993.

Gardner H. Are there additional intelligences? The case for naturalistic, spiritual and existential intelligences. In: Kane J, editor. *Education, Information and Transformation*. Upper Saddle River, NJ: Prentice Hall; 1999. pp. 111–31.

Goldberg LR. The structure of phenotypic personality traits. *American Psychologist*. 1993; **48**(1): 26–34.

Goleman D. *Emotional Intelligence: why it can matter more than IQ*. 10th ed. New York: Bantam Books; 1995.

Grewal D, Salovey P. Feeling smart: the science of emotional intelligence. *American Scientist*. 2005; **93**: 330–9.

Guleryuz G, Guney S, Aydn EM, *et al*. The mediating effect of job satisfaction between emotional intelligence and organisational commitment of nurses: a questionnaire survey. *Int J Nurs Stud*. 2008; **45**(11): 1625–35.

Hedlund J, Sternberg RJ. Practical intelligence: implications for human resources research. In: Ferris GR, editor. *Research in Personal and Human Resource Management*. Oxford: Elsevier Science; 2000.

Holmes C. The slow death of psychiatric nursing: what next? *J Psychiatr Ment Health Nurs*. 2006; **13**(4): 401–15.

Hunt T. The measurement of social intelligence. *J Appl Psychol*. 1928; **12**: 317–34.

Hurley J, Linsley P. Transformational leadership in neo-bureaucratic environments. *J Nurs Manag*. 2007; **15**: 749–55.

Limerick D, Cunnington B, Crowther F. *Managing the New Organisation: collaboration and sustainability in the post-corporate world*. 2nd ed. Crows Nest, NSW: Allen & Unwin; 2002.

Locke EA. Why emotional intelligence is an invalid concept. *J Organ Behavis*. 2005; **26**: 425–31.

Marlowe H. Social intelligence: evidence for multidimensionality and construct independence. *J Educ Psychol*. 1986; **78**(1), 52–8.

Mayer J. *Personality: a systems approach*. 3rd ed. Boston, MA: Pearsons; 2005.

Mayer J, Salovey P. What is emotional intelligence? In: Salovey P, Sluyter D, editors. *Emotional Development and Emotional Intelligence: implications for educators.* New York: Basic Books; 1997. pp. 3–31.

Mayer J, Salovey P, Caruso D. Selecting a measure for emotional intelligence. In: Bar-On R, 2000, op. cit. pp. 320–4.

Mayer J, Salovey P, Caruso D. Emotional intelligence: theories, findings and implications. *Psychological Inquiry.* 2004; **15**(3): 197–215.

Mayer J, Salovey P, Caruso D. Emotional intelligence: new ability or eclectic traits? *Am Psychol.* 2008; **16**(6): 503–17.

O'Connell E. Therapeutic relationships in critical care nursing: a reflection on practice. *Nurs Crit Care.* 2008; **13**(3): 138–43.

Salovey P, Mayer J. Emotional intelligence. *Imagination, Cognition, and Personality.* 1990; **9**(3): 185–211.

Silberman M. *Peoplesmart: developing your interpersonal intelligence.* San Francisco, CA: Berrett-Koehler Publishers Inc.; 2000.

Sorrentino R, Nezlek J, Yasunaga S, *et al.* Uncertainty orientation and affective experiences: individual differences within and across cultures. *J Cross Cult Psychol.* 2008; **39**(2): 129–46.

Sternberg R. *Successful intelligence.* New York: Plume; 1997.

Sternberg R, Grigorenko E. Practical intelligence and its development. In: Bar-On, 2000, op. cit. pp. 215–43.

Strang R. Measures of social intelligence. *American Journal of Sociology.* 1930; **36**: 263–9.

Van Rooy D, Viswesvaran C, Pluta P. An evaluation of construct validity: what is this thing called emotional intelligence? *Human Performance.* 2005; **18**(4): 445–62.

Wilson S, Carryer J. Emotional competence and nursing education: a New Zealand study. *Nurs Prax N Z.* 2008; **24**(1): 36–47.

CHAPTER 2

Why emotional intelligence matters in health and social care

John Hurley and Charlie Stansfield

Chapter 1 hopefully responded to the question of 'What is EI?' However, a second and possibly equally important question is: 'Does EI have any relevance to being a health or social care professional?'

This chapter seeks to respond to this second question by placing EI firmly within the contexts of your roles. We will consider our question about the relevance of EI by exploring who we are: in other words, can we uncover any evidence that connects EI to the identity of the professions you are currently joining, or have joined.

We will explore the published views of others, examine findings from a recent research study and search for any connections within relevant health and social policy. Finally, we will have our first 'story from the field' which gives you the opportunity to explore for yourself the application of EI to the world of practice. Hopefully, by considering our question from such a varied range of sources we can make an informed judgment on the relevance of EI to your work and studies.

EMOTIONAL INTELLIGENCE AS BEING PART OF PROFESSIONAL IDENTITY

The idea of reflecting upon who or what we are may initially appear to be superficial; in essence, you may believe that you know yourself entirely and what it means to be a social worker, a nurse or a medical doctor. However, your professional identity is not only something totally separate from your personal identity, itself influenced by an ever-evolving array of genetic, experiential and cultural factors.

Gee (1999), a commentator on identity, forwards the view that there is a multiplicity of identities held by an individual. Central to this view of identity is that, while a fixed perceived view of self exists as a core identity, individuals also assume less central identities in response to the contexts of their lives. Consequently, you may simultaneously hold the identities of occupational therapist, wife and perhaps even netball star.

This increasingly complicated understanding of who we are is made potentially even more confusing when reflecting upon the thought that our personal and professional identities are not all unchanging over time (Howard 2006). While a permanent identity may refer to unchangeable characteristics such as ethnicity, other parts of ourselves alter over time in response to new social contexts (Eisenberg 2001). Finally, let us not forget that our professional and personal identities are in fact not entirely separate and distinct from each other. This multiplicity of ebbing and flowing individual identities suggests that self-awareness, accurate self-assessment and adaptability, all key features of EI, are required to inform us on our personal and professional development and identity.

Box 2.1   Social-based reflective activity: personal identity

- Make a list of six characteristics that you feel makes the most significant contribution to your personal identity – in essence, what makes you who you are.
- Ask a peer or trusted other to also make a list of what he or she thinks are the most significant parts of your personal identity.
- Finally, were there any differences between your list of six characteristics about yourself as a person and the list made by your peer or trusted other? Are they 'wrong' about you, or are you 'wrong' about yourself? Or can both be true, i.e. our identity is both who we are and what others see?

As in the last chapter, be very mindful of your emotions and thoughts as you undertake these exercises and critically reflect on any insights you gain.

Box 2.2   Professional-based reflective activity: professional identity

Herminia Ibarra's (2007) research into professional identity reveals three basic tasks in the transition of professionals to more senior roles: 1) observing role models to identify potential identities; 2) experimenting with provisional selves; and 3) evaluating experience against internal standards and external feedback. **Are these processes also involved in the formation of professional identity as students begin working in real work environments?** Regardless of whether you are already a qualified practitioner or a student, answer the following questions:

- list role models from your chosen profession and their characteristics. Role models can be those people put forward by your chosen profession or those people you admire and would want to emulate
- list ways in which you have sought to incorporate these characteristics into your own professional practice
- what 'internal standards' do you work to and would not compromise as part of your clinical practice?
- compare your findings with the EI capabilities outlined in Chapter 1.

EMOTIONAL INTELLIGENCE AS BEING A PART OF PROFESSIONAL ROLES: THE VIEWS OF OTHERS FROM THE LITERATURE

Undertaking a literature review is an incredibly effective way to obtain a picture of current thinking on a topic without having to go out and do research. Below are critiques of recent papers on EI and your professional roles. A little later you will be asked to undertake the web-based activity of exploring what is known as 'the grey literature' which is most commonly policy documents from departmental sources.

Weng (2008) and Weng *et al.* (2008) suggest that there is a link between EI and contemporary medical roles. They highlight that the Accreditation Council for Graduate Medical Education includes many EI capabilities, and that the council undertakes assessment of these capabilities. Additionally, EI capabilities are often assessed as entry and progression criteria throughout the training process. Indeed, in striving to evidence a link between EI and improved patient–doctor relationships, Weng *et al.* (2008) undertook a large study of 994 patients and 39 doctors. Findings suggested that patients had improved trust with doctors with higher EI. Stratton, *et al.* (2008) continue this theme of connecting EI capabilities to effective medical practice through having better patient relationships by establishing links between EI and communication. Varkey *et al.* (2009) also highlight EI capabilities within medical leadership as being very important through identifying a range of EI capabilities including communication and conflict resolution as contributing to successful medical leadership.

Medicine is far from being alone in establishing a link between EI and professional roles. Within occupational therapy there is recognition that the emotionally intelligent therapist can facilitate his or her patient's emotional adjustment and rehabilitation in responding to disability. Additionally, the case for EI within occupational therapy is distinctly put by McKenna (2007) who identifies that holistic and client-centred occupational therapy requires EI to respond to the client's emotional needs. Indeed the supporting and development of EI is identified as a significant occupational therapy intervention to help those with a range of disabilities. Gunvor and Gyllensten (2000) extend the connectivity of enabling patients and enhancing professional practice through EI into the field of physiotherapy. Improved clinical reasoning processes, better therapeutic relationships and enhanced health communication are all cited as the main advantages for physiotherapy practice. The social work profession has also acknowledged EI as being an enabling construct for social workers to take on and seek to resolve social problems and be effective leaders (Burgess 2005).

While all health and social work professions identify EI as being an integral to their roles, it is nursing that has the widest range of literature exploring this link.

EI has long been identified as being important to nursing. Öhlén and Segesten (1998), who specifically researched nurse identity, found links between EI and professional nurse identity. Self-knowledge, stress tolerance and professional knowledge as well as trust in one's own capacity and feelings were all raised by nurse participants in the study as significant factors in their personal/professional identity. Freshwater and Stickley (2004) highlight EI as being an essential capability to engage in effective nursing roles. Such is the relevance of EI to nursing that authors such as Cadman and Brewer (2001) suggest that EI measures should be used for the selection of nursing candidates.

More recently, Mikolajczak, Menil and Luminet (2007) demonstrate through their study that EI traits are highly effective protective factors in stressful environments. In their study of over 100 nurses, those with high levels of EI traits showed markedly lower levels of stress or somatic problems. Rydon (2005) found that self-knowledge is an essential capability for engaging effectively with therapeutic relating while Davies *et al.* (2010) identify EI as underpinning district nurse practice. Austin *et al.* (2007) identified empathy as being central in achieving effective healthcare delivery while Wilson and Carryer (2008) linked a nurse's fitness to practice to his or her having EI capabilities.

EMOTIONAL INTELLIGENCE AS BEING A PART OF PROFESSIONAL ROLES: THE VIEWS OF OTHERS FROM POLICIES

For many, policy is something to refer to when seeking clarification regarding a matter or concern of practice. While this may have some truth, it is also inescapable that policy shapes our day-to-day roles, determines education programmes and influences our professional identity. In short, if policy links EI to your work roles, then it must have some relevance.

Most countries and many states will have policies detailing the capabilities they see as being essential for their health and social care workforce. Of interest to us is if these capabilities reflect in any way those of the EI models detailed in Chapter 1, Introducing emotional intelligence.

Box 2.3   Web-based activity

Conduct a search of recent policies pertinent to your geographical region and discipline. Focus on major policies and documents which look at the capabilities of the workforce or capabilities needed to provide high standards of care.

You may also wish to look beyond the limits of geography and discipline to see what is happening elsewhere. The 'publications' section of health and social service government department websites are good starting places.

EMOTIONAL INTELLIGENCE AS BEING A PART OF PROFESSIONAL ROLES: THE VIEWS TAKEN DIRECTLY FROM NURSES

The literature review and the search of policies (often referred to as grey literature) should be building a picture that indicates relevance exists between EI capabilities and being capable within your chosen profession. However, is there any evidence that professionals working within the field are also saying something similar? This section presents findings of a qualitative study by Hurley (2009) exploring this very question of links between EI and professional roles.

The study of 24 nurses in England and Scotland was structured around social constructionism that focuses on how language used within social contexts and relationships builds understandings (Berger and Luckmann 1966, Gergen 1999). A direct phenomenological approach that focuses upon human conscious knowing and shared meanings among participants was assumed for the study (Titchen and Hobson 2005).

Goleman's EI model highlights the relational aspect between the self and others that has been shown as central to nursing (Hurley and Rankin 2008). Consequently, findings from the study are organised in relation to the four broad areas of EI outlined in Chapter 1, Introducing Emotional Intelligence (Consortium for Research on Emotional Intelligence in Organisations 1998). Table 2.1 shows the percentage of respondents in each participant category who identified that EI quadrant as being important to nursing.

Generally, the participants communicated a high value toward personal recognition and social regulation EI capabilities as being central to their roles. This use of the personal self within professional helping roles is well-established (Peplau 1989, p. 28; Barker 2000). Interestingly, the data showed a greater focus by the female participants on all aspects of EI; females have previously been noted as having a higher awareness than men of their own emotions and the emotions of others (Humple, Caputi and Martin 2001).

TABLE 2.1 EI capabilities identified as being important to the effective helping of others

Categories	Personal recognition	Personal regulation	Social recognition	Social regulation
Academic	100%	50%	50%	100%
Clinical	88%	65%	76%	82%
Managerial	67%	100%	33%	67%
Male	82%	64%	64%	73%
Female	93%	69%	69%	93%

> **Box 2.4**   Reflective activity
>
> Read the themes and quotes from the participants below and reflect upon their views. Do you agree that your professional role requires these capabilities?
>
> Keep these capabilities and quotes in mind as you read Charlie Stansfield's story from clinical practice that follows.

The themes found in the study were:

Theme 1. Knowing yourself

Personal recognition (92% of participants) – Participants identified the following capabilities as being central to their nursing roles:

- emotional self-awareness
- accurate self-assessment
- self-confidence.

Research Participant (RP) 3: *'Self-awareness is massive; it's impossible to see how someone could be a good mental health nurse without an essential grasp of themselves … how they feel about people. I think learning values are embedded in self-awareness as well, understanding how you feel, how you come across, how other people might judge you, so yes I see there is a very strong link between being person-centred, recognising people, recognising yourself, managing interactions well through social skills and emotional regulation. I see there is an intrinsic link between all of these things.'*

Theme 2. Helping others

Social regulation (87% of participants) – Participants identified the following relationship management capabilities as being pivotal to their roles:

- developing others
- influence
- communication
- conflict management.

RP15: *'Giving people back their responsibility – I think that's really important. You can provide them with the right tools, and I know it doesn't always work and people don't always want to take that responsibility, but I think you've got to. I think if they want to you've got to try and keep them motivated and support them to make the right choices.'*

Theme 3. Managing yourself

Personal regulation (71% of participants) – Participants identified the following self-management capabilities as being central:

- trustworthiness
- adaptability
- achievement drive.

RP25: *'I seem to be going back to the mentality that yeah, emotional self-awareness is very important. Self-control … being aware of emotions, it's not enough. They need to be able to effectively regulate emotions when you are working with somebody so that your own emotions aren't spilling out onto the relationship of the service user. I think you need to be trustworthy as well and I suppose [have] adaptability.'*

Theme 4. Acknowledging others

Social recognition (71% of participants) – Participants identified the following social awareness capabilities as being central to mental health nurses' (MHNs) engaging with talk-based therapies:

- empathy
- service orientation
- organisational awareness.

RP12: *'Empathy is definitely one that you have, and need to have …. Your empathy doesn't trigger some kind of rescuing response where you can jump in and save the day and get the credit for it …. At the end of the day you can help this person; you can help them become better at being themselves.'*

APPLYING EMOTIONAL INTELLIGENCE: STORIES FROM THE FIELD

It is often the case that interest and conviction about the relevance of a theory come alive when connection is made with lived experience. The following scenario is a true story, with obvious details changed.

Lou's bed is in a room with three others at the end of a long corridor. The place was built in the 1940s, its beige walls are peeling in places and scuffed. At one end of the corridor, a man in his pyjama bottoms sits on a plastic chair by a payphone, shouting into the handset.

As I walk down to Lou's room, I pass two nurses struggling on either side of an older man, who is having difficulty standing without aid. One nurse wears a plastic apron. It is close to lunchtime, the institutional smell of boiled vegetables hangs in the air.

Lou, who has been a straight-A student for most of her life, is sitting on her bed in tracksuit pants and a t-shirt, with textbooks spread around her. Until recently, she was scoring high-distinctions for most of her law degree assignments. Now, Lou is being 'specialled'. This means she has one nurse with her at all times. One of them reports that Lou spends mealtimes cutting each food item on her plate into tiny segments and then mixing them all together. By the time the allocated time for meals is over, she has eaten very little. The nurse records what she actually eats, then escorts and supervises the compulsory bed rest, which follows each meal.

'Get me out of here', she says, handing me a piece of paper. 'I can't eat this crap.' The menu she hands me lists a variety of high-fat, high-sugar foods supplemented by Sustagen.

We go outside to a balcony where a group of other patients are sitting in silence, smoking. The Eating Disorder Unit, mainly young women, shares its space with an adult psychiatric ward, mainly dishevelled-looking older men. The ill-matched group sits together on plastic chairs with overflowing ashtrays by their feet and cans of diet coke on the table.

I give Lou the cigarettes she has asked for; she looks around furtively, and takes the pack. She lights one up from the stub offered by a man sitting beside us. She picks at the faint scars on her arm as we talk. Lou says she is willing to eat but only wants to eat what she considers to be healthy foods. Fruit, vegetables and little else. Anything more substantial terrifies her. She's been told if she doesn't follow the menu as depicted on the diet sheet, she will have to undergo a nasogastric tube feed. She has been on the ward for four days and has refused to follow the menu, despite having a nurse sit watching her as she eats. Her showers are supervised and a nurse stands outside the door of the toilet. Lou weights about 43 kilos. Her body mass index (BMI) is under 20. She points out, given weight and height ratios, that Nicole Kidman's BMI must be about the same.

Lou tells me she hates being in hospital, but does acknowledge she has been unwell. She says she feels she is in prison, her every movement watched.

'If you asked for a salad for lunch no one would object', she says, 'but if I do, it's just another symptom of my anorexic thinking'.

I'm there to attend the weekly ward round as an observer. The professor responsible for the Eating Disorders Unit chairs it. He is a rotund psychiatrist in his early 60s. He looks like he hasn't had time to get dressed properly, the buttons on his stained shirt are done up all wrong. He has a cup of black coffee by his side, and a file full of papers that he rifles through while everyone sits in silence, waiting.

He opens the case discussion about Lou by quoting statistics about anorexia nervosa and refers to Lou as 'a chronic case' with poor prognosis. It is her first admission to this hospital, but she has been on other hospital treatment programs in the past. The nursing unit manager (NUM) reads from a file and tells the group that Lou is non-compliant and manipulative. I ask what the evidence is for the latter. She looks up from her clipboard and states that Lou had agreed to follow the program and undertake no exercise, but was later observed jogging in the shower.

The dietician speaks next. She likens Lou to the others on the ward in that she is 'preoccupied with cleansing detox diets and veganism, and won't comply with the menu set'. The whippet-thin dietician jigs while she talks and taps her pen on her files when others talk. She notes that Lou, like a lot of people with anorexia, has obsessively studied nutrition and seems to be trying to survive on the absolute bare minimum. She says her last consultation with Lou lasted for an hour as Lou insisted on debating the pros and cons of soy milk. The dietician says she just doesn't have time for this, but that she felt manipulated into the conversation.

The professor nods at the trainee psychiatrist, a young man staring out of the window. Jolted out of his daydream he suggests a possible increase in Lou's anti-depressant medication. An intern psychologist states Lou's file refers to a history of sexual abuse. The social worker mentions that 'the family live in an affluent suburb and the father has visited briefly'. Another nurse says she has had to remove Weight Watchers magazines from underneath Lou's mattress. She also says she is tired of the 'circular' conversations with Lou, where she won't accept her goal weight.

I ask if anyone has had a chance to discuss Lou's own goals for this treatment program with her. I mention that she can't be kept in hospital against her will forever so she needs to be working towards some sort of plan. It seems unnecessary to point out the gulf of understanding between Lou and the treatment team as to what constitutes her good health. The psychologist states he is only on the ward for one day a week and Lou said she didn't want to see him. The nursing unit manager (NUM) says that they 'don't plan with any of the girls until they have gained some weight'.

The discussion turns back to the menu and the calorific intake. They talk again about a nasogastric tube feed as a last resort if she continues to refuse to eat. The bed-search nurse says, 'I think we should lay it on the line, she either eats what's on the menu or she has a nasogastric feed. It's really just about a battle of wills'.

The professor nods at me but nobody else says anything. He says, 'Well we ought to get her in and see what she has to say'.

I ask if those who are not directly responsible for Lou's program need to be present. I point out that this is a large group of people and might be intimidating for Lou. There are about 15 professionals in the room all sitting around a long table, some of whom are there to talk about other patients, not Lou. The professor nods. Several nurses get up and shuffle out. The psychologist picks up his papers and leaves reluctantly.

Lou appears at the door, skinny and pale. She sits on the edge of a chair. The professor asks her how she is, and she says in a tiny, childlike voice that she hates the hospital and wants to go home and get back to Uni.

'It's not working', Lou says. 'It's not going to work'.

He asks her to speak up.

She repeats herself in a marginally louder voice.

There's tension in the air. The NUM snaps, 'Lou, you know the situation here, you've done this before, you need to comply with the program'. The rest of the ward round look at Lou.

The prof says she can go home when she has reached her goal weight about four kilos away. Lou interrupts to question the goal weight. He talks about the effect of not eating on her heart, brain and cognitive function, and stresses how important it is for her to eat the foods the dietician has proposed.

Lou has tuned out. She stares at her feet. He tells her if there isn't any progress within the next few days then they will have to look at a nasogastric feed. He asks her if she has any questions. She looks up and asks in barely audible tones whether half the weight he has suggested would suffice. The NUM sighs and looks at the ceiling. The prof smiles. 'We will review how you are going and we can discuss this again next ward round in a week's time'. Lou blurts out, 'A week?' As she stands up to leave, a nurse jumps up and stands beside her. 'We will get you well and then you can go home', the prof says firmly. Lou is escorted out of the meeting.

'I think the nasogastric is going to be the only option', the NUM says. 'She's very stubborn, very entrenched, it's going to start affecting the other girls.'

I later talk with Lou about her options. She complains about the program and when I ask her what she thinks would improve it, she thinks for a moment, and then says, 'Love!'

The final activity for you to undertake in this chapter is from Charlie Stansfield's story and poses incredibly complex questions and reflections. Underneath the activity questions lay deeper issues of differing perspectives toward truth and reality, patient and staff all being under incredible emotional strain and the mutual use of power to control others, as well as the potential of empathy to be a crucial mitigating EI capability. An important consideration when undertaking the activity is to reflect upon how the ability to assume the other's perspective could impact upon his or her actions. Revisit the EI capabilities outlined in any model in Chapter 1 and imaginatively apply these to all participants in the story.

Box 2.5 Social-based activity

What is striking is the difficult position the treatment team in the previous story is placed in, having to obviously ensure that people don't become so under-weight that their health is seriously threatened, but also to forge a genuine therapeutic relationship with someone like Lou, who is clearly in a tortuous position. Somehow the treatment team and Lou need to work together. In pairs or small groups, respond to the following.

Focus on using EI capabilities:
- if you were working on the ward described, detail some of the simple things you could do to try to improve the experience of patients
- look at the staff within this story. What EI capabilities were or were not being communicated and what would you do that is different? What EI capabilities would help Lou and how would you go about helping her develop them?

CONCLUSION

We commenced this brief chapter with a question: 'Does EI have any relevance to being a health or social care professional?' We have explored the views of others through published academic papers, policy and a story from the field of practice.

Certainly, EI does not make up the entirety of personal or professional roles, but it does arguably make up important aspects of these roles, and hence our professional identities. Through understanding the relevance of EI to the successful undertaking of our professional roles we are also alerted to the importance of developing not only our academic and clinical skills and capabilities, but also the capabilities grouped under the term of EI.

REFERENCES

Austin E, Evans P, Magnus B, *et al*. A preliminary study of empathy, emotional intelligence and examination performance in MBChB students. *Med Educ.* 2007; **41**(7): 684–9.

Barker P. The tidal model: the lived experience in person-centred mental health care. *Nursing Philosophy.* 2000; **2**(3): 213–23.

Berger P, Luckmann T. *The Social Construction of Reality.* London: Penguin Books; 1966.

Burgess R. A model for enhancing individual and organisational learning of 'emotional intelligence': the drama and winner's triangles. *Social Work Education.* 2005; **24**(1): 97–112.

Cadman C, Brewer J. Emotional intelligence: a vital ingredient for recruitment in nursing. *J Nurs Manag.* 2001; **9**: 321–4.

Consortium for Research on Emotional Intelligence in Organizations. *Emotional competence framework.* 1998. Available at: www.eiconsortium.org/reports/emotional_competence_framework.html (accessed 17 July 2011).

Davies S, Jenkins E, Mabbett G. Emotional intelligence: district nurses' lived experiences. *Br J Community Nurs.* 2010; **15**(3): 141–6.

Department of Health. *Commissioning a Brighter Future: improving access to psychological therapies.* London: Department of Health; 2007.

Eisenberg E. Building a mystery: toward a new theory of communication and identity. *J Commun.* 2001; **51**: 534–52.

Freshwater D, Stickley T. The heart of the art: emotional intelligence in nurse education. *Nursing Inquiry.* 2004; **11**(2): 91–8.

Gee J. *An introduction to Discourse Analysis: theory and method.* London and New York: Routledge; 1999.

Gergen K. *An Invitation to Social Construction.* London: Sage Publications; 1999.

Gunvor G, Gyllensten A. The importance of emotions in physiotherapeutic practice. *Physical Therapy Reviews.* 2000; **5**(3): 155–60.

Howard J. Expecting and accepting: the temporal ambiguity of recovery identities. *Soc Psychol Q.* 2006; **69**(4): 307–24.

Humple N, Caputi P, Martin C. The relationship between emotions and stress among mental health nurses. *Australian and New Zealand Journal of Mental Health Nursing.* 2001; **10**(1), 55–60.

Hurley J. A qualitative study of mental health nurse identities: many roles, one profession. *Int J Ment Health Nurs.* 2009; **18**: 383–90.

Hurley J, Rankin R. As mental health nursing roles expand is education expanding mental health nurses? An emotionally intelligent view toward preparation for psychological therapies and relatedness. *Nurs Inq.* 2008; **15**(3): 199–205.

Ibarra H. *Working Identity: unconventional strategies for reinventing your career.* Boston, MA: Harvard Business School Press; 2007.

Mikolajczak M, Menil C, Luminet O. Explaining the protective effect of trait emotional intelligence regarding occupational stress: exploration of emotional labour processes. *Journal of Research in Personality.* 2007; **41**: 1107–17.

McKenna J. Emotional intelligence training in adjustment to physical disability and illness. *International Journal of Therapy & Rehabilitation.* 2007; **14**(12): 551–6.

Öhlén J, Segesten K. The professional identity of the nurse: concept analysis and development. *J Adv Nurs.* 1998; **28**(4): 720–7.

Peplau HE. Theory: the professional dimension. In: O'Toole A, Welt S, editors. *Interpersonal Theory in Nursing Practice: selected works of Hildegard E. Peplau.* New York: Springer; 1989. pp. 21–30.

Rydon SE. The attitudes, knowledge and skills needed in mental health nurses: the perspective of users of mental health services. *Int J Ment Health Nurs.* 2005; **14**: 78–87.

Stratton TD, Saunders JA, Elam CL. Changes in medical students' emotional intelligence: an exploratory study. *Teach Learn Med.* 2008; **20**(3): 279–84.

Titchen A, Hobson D. Phenomenology. In: Somekh B, Lewin C, editors. *Research Methods in the Social Sciences.* London: Sage Publications; 2005. pp. 121–30.

Varkey P, Peloquin J, Reed D, *et al.* Leadership curriculum in undergraduate medical education: a study of student and faculty perspectives. *Med Teach.* 2009; **31**(3): 244–50.

Weng H. Does the physician's emotional intelligence matter? Impacts of the physician's emotional intelligence on the trust, patient-physician relationship, and satisfaction. *Health Care Manage Rev.* 2008; **33**(4): 280–8.

Weng HC, Chen HC, Chen HJ, *et al.* Doctors' emotional intelligence and the patient-doctor relationship. *Med Educ.* 2008; **42**(7): 703–11.

Wilson S, Carryer J. Emotional competence and nursing education: a New Zealand study. *Nurs Prax N Z.* 2008; **24**(1): 36–47.

CHAPTER 3

Self-awareness and empathy: foundational skills for practitioners

John Hurley, Paul Linsley and Charlie Stansfield

This chapter focuses upon self-awareness and empathy as being foundational EI capabilities and seeks to clarify what both of these terms mean. Arguably, without self-awareness and the capability of recognising the needs of others, our health- and social-based interventions are significantly less effective. Additionally, our ability to work and get on with others in team and work units is connected to our ability to accurately perceive aspects of self, and of other people. IQ alone will not be enough to be completely effective in either of these work areas. Hence, this chapter explores a variety of approaches to understanding and potentially enhancing self-awareness and empathy.

You will recall from Chapter 1, Introducing Emotional Intelligence, that Gardner (1993, 1999), Salovey and Mayer (1990), Bar-On (2000) and Goleman (1995) all included the capabilities of self-awareness and empathy into their models of intelligence. Given the areas of dispute and disagreement between these researchers this unanimous inclusion of self-awareness and empathy communicates the importance of both of these capabilities. While having different interpretations and emphasis towards self-awareness and empathy, these authors variously described self-awareness and empathy as:

- being able to perceive emotions in oneself and others accurately
- the ability to understand emotions
- the ability to understand emotional language
- the ability to understand the signals conveyed by emotions
- being aware of and understanding our emotions
- knowing which emotions we are feeling and why.

REALITY

Without becoming diverted into a philosophical debate on the nature of humanity, there is worth in very briefly considering self-awareness and empathy from a broad perspective. Considering these core EI capabilities without at least offering a passing thought to the fabric of the reality in which we view ourselves and others would remove the very context in which they are enacted.

In seeking to grasp an understanding of the nature of knowledge, being and ultimately ourselves, humanity has contemplated and embraced varied philosophical viewpoints. Dualism, whereby an internal conscious self simultaneously exists with the external world, is the view toward our human existence that underpins Western modernism (Gergen 1999). However, how can we be certain that the information acquired from the external world has been accurately registered in our internal world of self? Alternatively, all of reality could be understood in the belief that nothing exists outside the mind, effectively describing human experience as being nothing more or less than an individual projection.

Yet another approach called critical realism presumes there are in fact two realities in which we dwell. The first being the relatively constant physical reality and the second being the reality we perceive (Pawson and Tilley 1997). An example of how self, others and reality may be perceived in a very different way can be found in something called social constructionism. Here reality is considered to be built from the shared understandings between people. An example of this might be how physical beauty varies with cultural and over time (Gergen 2001).

Antagonistic debate on the differing realities offers little progression on our task of understanding self-awareness and empathy better. However, being aware of the diversity of the ways we can understand the nature of reality and hence ourselves and others shows our task is perhaps not as straightforward as might be initially imagined.

SELF-AWARENESS

Arguably, it is the understanding of the origins of our thoughts and emotions and those of others that offers the greatest challenge. This can be true both for our professional roles and within our personal lives.

Box 3.1 Reflective activity

Ask yourself the following question: If knowing yourself in totality equals a score of 10 out of 10 for being self-aware, and a score of zero out of 10 equals a score of being totality self-unaware, what score out of 10 would you honestly allocate yourself?

It has been the authors' experience over many years that when most groups are asked this question, they average out at around seven out of 10. Indeed it is extremely rare for anyone to forward a 10 out of 10 score, even when the scoring is done confidentially. Given this, there is a very important question to reflect upon. If I know what 70% or even 80% of me is doing, feeling and/or thinking at any given time, what is the other 30% or 20% of me up to? The answer may sometimes lay in often heard phrases such as: 'Why did I say that; why did I go out with him; how did I end up doing this course' or incidents when we find ourselves wishing for a time machine to go back and rectify a comment, action or a poorly communicated view.

Box 3.2   Reflective activity

In Chapter 2 you were asked, amongst other things, to make a list of six characteristics that you believe make the most significant contribution to your personal identity – in essence what makes you who you are. Now consider the following.

- How did you reach your decisions to populate that list?
- How did these characteristics about you come into being?
- Were there significant discrepancies between your view of yourself and the view of the trusted other? If so, is this your restricted self-awareness, or their restricted empathic understanding of you?

Self-awareness is important for staff to master since it allows them to develop, reflect and learn from experiences, as well as to be able to identify obstacles that could hinder the care that they provide for patients. Within a modern, Western-orientated context, self-awareness is most frequently dominated by cognitive reflection, with the emotional self relegated to a secondary identity, and the spiritual self often unconsidered (Hurley 2008, Pfeifer and Cox 2007). This narrowing of ways of understanding ourselves and others arguably fails to respond to the required full-depth human engagement, hence often culminating in stressful and disharmonious human relations, resulting in conflicting needs and values (Szasz 1983, pp. 21, 23). So what might this 'self' that we are to be aware of actually be? Montgomery (1997) suggested that clinical staff members are reluctant to deal with emotional states such as anxiety and depression because they lack the necessary understanding and skills to deal with them completely. Moreover, staff may avoid situations that mirror experiences within their own personal lives, which could result in avoidance behaviour that they are not aware of.

Self can at its most basic level be understood as being the totality of what we are within the boundary of our physical bodies (Perls *et al.* 1973). However, we (self) then interact with our surrounding physical environment and hence have new experiences. These experiences in turn may (or may not) change some small or even possibly significant part of our selves. As discussed in Chapter 2, the self (and hence others around us) comprise a complex mix through having some permanence and yet also changing with new experiences. An example of this is that we may, to varying degrees, separate or integrate our personal and professional selves. This in turn tells us that we (and those around us) choose which parts of self to adopt and which parts to repress. This split between adoption and repression in itself requires self-awareness to make that choice, and then of course the authenticity to avoid self-deception. Consequently, when we are relating with other people it is often a meeting of two people sharing certain parts of themselves whilst hiding other parts.

Jung (1928) first introduced the concept of the persona, or masks that humans adopt as we undertake our social roles, and it is his work that alerts us to the dangers of self-deception. Our social roles (for example: nurse, friend, parent) are mainly in step with our true 'inner self', allowing an emotional ease and fluid behaviours within our adopted personas (nurse, friend and parent), and these personas are mutually understood by those around us. However, these different personas within us can also be in conflict, or the inner self become lost within the multiplicity of adopted masks.

A core consideration is consequently how to reach a level of self-awareness that allows us to see ourselves more completely and honestly. Additionally, if understanding ourselves is a challenging undertaking, how difficult then is it to be truly empathic toward another complex, multiple and partially changing other?

A firm understanding and acceptance of self allows the carer to acknowledge a patient's differences and uniqueness. Campbell (1980) has identified a holistic model of self-awareness that consists of four interconnected components: psychological, physical, environmental and philosophical.

- The **psychological component** includes knowledge of emotions, motivations, self-concept and personality. Being psychologically self-aware means being sensitive to feelings and to external elements that affect those feelings.
- The **physical component** is the knowledge of personal and general physiology, as well as of bodily sensations, body image and physical potential.
- The **environmental component** consists of the sociocultural environment, relationships with others, and knowledge of the relationship between humans and nature.
- The **philosophical component** is the sense of life having meaning. A personal philosophy of life and death may or may not include a superior being but does take into account responsibility to the world and the ethics of behaviour.

Together these components provide a model that can be used to promote the self-awareness and self-growth of providers and those they care for.

Let us first overview different approaches that may help us be more self-aware before undertaking some exercises in self-awareness.

While being far from an all-inclusive overview of ways to challenge our current levels of self-awareness, the following offer a good foundational understanding of self-awareness processes. A word of caution is offered in adopting one approach of understanding self and others to the exclusion of all others; experiential psychology and spirituality as outlined below all offer potential paths to explore and enhance self-awareness (Hurley 2008).

Cognitive behavioural psychology

Modern psychology places great emphasis upon cognition dictating behaviour, arguably at the expense of other aspects of self (Ehrich 2003). Amongst the varied approaches within mainstream psychology, the cognitive behavioural view is enjoying a remarkable rise in popularity. This view proposes that people have a schema or map of themselves, the world and the future, which is formed from real-life experiences and attempts to impose meaning upon life events (Beech 2000). Automatic thoughts and self-statements generated by our personal schemata directly influence our emotional responses, and consequently our behaviours. Values are placed upon thoughts by ourselves and those around us as being rational or irrational and emotions as either positive or negative. Self-knowledge and change focuses upon knowing and subsequently altering our faulty life schemata. This cognitive behavioural view of the self boldly claims to be capable of valid, reliable and accurate empirical measurement of human subjective experiences whilst maintaining an overarching framework of humanistic principles (Beech 2000).

Box 3.3 Reflective activity

In words or through drawing images, express what your core schemata is for the three points below. Be much more detailed in your responses than the examples offered. When completed reflect upon how these beliefs direct your emotions and how you conduct yourself in your daily life.

Q1 What are your true beliefs about yourself?

Example answer: I am essentially an intelligent and hard person who is vulnerable to nobody.

Q2 What are your true beliefs about others?

Example answer: People are fundamentally out for what they can get off you, so get them before they get you.

Q3 What are your core beliefs about your immediate world?

Example answer: Everyone is a fool until proven otherwise.

Experiential psychology

In contrast to cognitive behavioural approaches, existential psychology places primacy upon an experiential rather than a cognitive self (Clarkson 1989, p. 13). More congruent with phenomenological philosophy rather than biological models, the self is seen as an integration of physical body, intellect and feelings, as well as perceptions within a social environment. Perceiving, feeling and behaviour are phenomenologically undertaken, rather than the emphasis being upon re-scribing existing schemata. One way of highlighting the differences between this approach and that of cognitive behavioural approaches is that the experiential-phenomenological approach prizes a journey of self-discovery led by curiosity driven questions concerning 'what is going on here?' This phenomenological approach allows a stepping aside from habitual thinking patterns, subsequently allowing potential for enhanced existential perception of both self and the external environment (Idhe 1977, cited in Yontef 1993). Consequently, both subjective feelings and objective observations are considered to have real meaning (Hurley 2008). Alternatively, the cognitive behavioural approaches prize a journey of self-discovery led by attaining pre-determined goals.

Box 3.4   Reflective activity

How you experience and make sense of different emotional states is an important element in emotional intelligence and reflective practice. Answer the three challenging questions below; do you feel uncomfortable in answering them?

Q1 What do you experience when reflecting on your true belief about yourself?

Example answer: I feel nothing; I don't allow myself to feel as I only pay attention to what I think.

Q2 What do you experience when reflecting on your true beliefs about others?

Example answer: I feel safe and I feel good about myself.

Q3 What are your core beliefs about your immediate world?

Example answer: I feel lonely.

Spirituality

Our spiritual selves are not frequently considered when engaged in reflection, particularly within professional and academically focused activity. However, spirituality may be seen as something that goes beyond constituting a broad faith to include the values and ethics by which we conduct ourselves (Hurley 2008). Within the field of health and social care this may include ethical models such as virtue ethics and emphasising the emotional self within decision-making (Cox *et al.* 2007, pp. 20–21). Clarity toward our own values necessitates self-knowledge to direct our actions and self perceptions, particularly when confronted with major decision-making, a time when established values can be challenged (Atwell and Fulford 2007, p. 90). When considering that significant power differentials exist between practitioners and those they are helping, an awareness of values appears vital.

Spiritual models of self-construct identify self-concept as the totality of the individual's thoughts and feelings, creating a subjective phenomena originating from and continually influenced by social experience (Bhugra 2007, p. 126). This self incorporates factors such as gender, social roles and ideology, as well as the physical self, personality and external input by others. These characteristics are bound by systemic senses of self-moral worth, self-determination, unity and competence (Gordon as cited by Bhugra 2007, pp. 128–9).

Box 3.5   Reflective activity

While modern psychology approaches make claim to activities that enhance self-awareness it must be remembered that spiritual approaches precede these by many thousands of years. Mindfulness, now a common intervention in psychological therapies and development workshops, has roots in Buddhism and Hinduism, to name but two such approaches.

Take a mindful walk, clearing your mind of thoughts and being open to the sensory stimuli coming into you. Be aware of thoughts and feeling that emerge into your awareness as you do this; do not try to suppress them, simply be aware of them and release them so you can then be open to the next sensory experience. Some may find this easy, others not. Keep practising this in increasingly challenging environments which are not quite so peaceful or quiet.

Ask yourself: Where do these emerging thoughts and feelings come from? Are you constantly aware of them? What might be the implications if you are not?

Becoming self-aware

Based on the above, self-awareness is the process of understanding one's own beliefs, thoughts, motivations, biases, and physical and emotional limitations and recognising how they affect others with whom we interact. The basic EI paradigm, which all the main schools mentioned in Chapter 1, broadly comprises four domains (Morrison 2007) (*see* Figure 3.1).

There are two intrapersonal domains: self-awareness and self-management, and two interpersonal domains: awareness of others/empathy and relationship skills. The arrows indicate the interrelationships that exist between all four domains. The arrows also indicate the interrelatedness across the four domains, particularly between self-awareness and empathy for others as a basis for managing self and relationships (Morrison 2007). Shulman (1999, p. 156) encapsulates the relevance of this for practitioners when he states: 'The capacity to be in touch with the client's feelings is related to the worker's ability to acknowledge his/

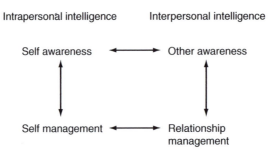

FIGURE 3.1 The basic EI paradigm

her own. Before a worker can understand the power of emotion in the life of the client, it is necessary to discover its importance in the worker's own experience'.

Self-awareness in the contexts of EI and being an effective health and social care practitioner is about knowing what you are thinking and feeling at any given moment. It is then about being able to ensure that your thoughts and emotions are productively focused on the key work at hand, and that your thoughts and emotions are working in harmony to achieve these ends. Given that this is not an easy task, even in environments supportive to self-awareness, this task is made more difficult given the challenging contexts of health and social care work. Naturally, these health and social care contexts inevitably include working with other people, necessitating the capacity for empathy.

No one can ever completely be self-aware; there is always something that is not known to us, and something waiting to be discovered. A much quoted and often cited model of self-awareness is the Johari Window. This information processing model was developed by the American psychologists Joseph Luft and Harry Ingham in the 1950s, calling it 'Johari' after combining their first names, Joe and Harry. The model emphasises the importance of reflection and self-analysis through the use of a 'window' (*see* Figure 3.2 *below*).

Each quadrant, or windowpane, describes one aspect of self. Each windowpane also contains and represents information. **Quadrant 1** is the open quadrant; this is what is known by the person about themselves and is also known to others. It includes the behaviours, feelings and thoughts known to the individual and

1 Known to self and others	2 Known only to others
3 Known only to self	4 Known neither to self nor others

FIGURE 3.2 The Johari Window

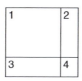

FIGURE 3.3 The Johari Window showing someone who can claim to be self-aware

shared and accessible by others. **Quadrant 2** is called the 'blind self' or 'blind spot', as it contains all the things that others know but the individual does not know. **Quadrant 3** is the hidden self or avoided self; it includes all the things that the person knows about him- or herself that others do not know. **Quadrant 4** is the unknown quadrant or unknown self, containing aspects of the self unknown to the individual and to others. No one ever completely knows his or her inner self, but sometimes we catch glimpses of it. It is like walking into a darkened room that you have not been in before and switching a torch on and off, catching sights that may be familiar but at the same time surprising. Taken together, the quadrants represent the total self.

The goal of increasing self-awareness is to enlarge the area of Quadrant 1 while reducing the size of the other three quadrants (*see* Figure 3.3). A reduction in Quadrant 2 is achieved through listening to and learning from others. Knowledge of self is not possible alone. As we relate to others, we broaden our perceptions of self, but learning requires active listening and openness to the feedback others provide. A reduction in Quadrant 3 is brought about by self-disclosing, or revealing to others important aspects of self.

Important within the construct of self-awareness is the process of personal experience. Although the individual might be open to feedback and comment from others, subjective responses will come into play in the interpretation of this information. Suspending judgement on self and responding instead to the evidence provided by others can be difficult and at times painful.

What aspects of self should we explore?

An important question in the pursuit of self-awareness is: what aspects of self should we seek to focus on and change? Fortunately, an exhaustive list of self aspects has been put forward (*see* Ben-Artzi *et al*. 1995) and incorporated into a diagram below (*see* Figure 3.4).

Important here is to recognise that self-awareness involves knowing that we are the same person across time (self-history), that we are the author of our thoughts and actions and that we are distinct from our environment (Kircher and David 2003); that we are an independent and unique entity in the world. Whilst we cannot control the actions and thoughts of others we can take responsibility for our own behaviour.

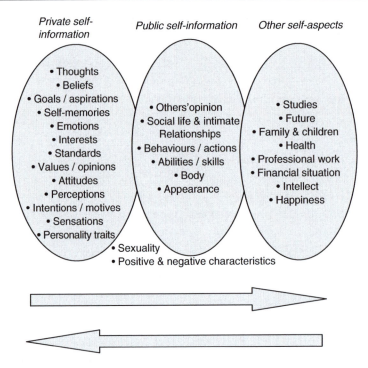

FIGURE 3.4 Aspects of self-awareness

EMPATHY

There are many ways of understanding what the term empathy means. Within the context of this book, we are adopting the view that empathy is the ability or capability that allows us to do the following:[*]

- to identify emotions in other people
- to interpret the meanings that emotions convey in others
- to monitor emotions in relation to others
- to manage emotion in others (Mayer and Salovey 1997)
- to be aware of and understanding how others feel (Bar-On 2000)
- to be able to show sensitivity and understand others' perspectives
- to be able to understand the perspective of others (Goleman 1995).

The above list may initially appear to sound a little impersonal by describing empathy as an ability and capability. However, this becomes warmer if you reflect upon what exactly the above list of abilities means. Empathy is in effect being able to have an understanding of what another person is experiencing and then respectfully apply that understanding to the context you and the other person are currently sharing.

---

[*] Naturally, empathy is only effective for the other person when our awareness of understanding and sensitivity is communicated to the other person.

Perhaps the best way to understand empathy is to take a moment and undertake the activity below.

Box 3.6 Social-based activity

Choose a partner to do this exercise with. Now choose a real experience you have had in life, an experience that was emotional for you and that has impacted upon you in a meaningful way. Tell that story to your partner, but leave out any details about what you felt at the time or how the event affected you. At various stages of your story ask your partner what they think you might have been feeling and thinking at the time.

(This can also be an exercise in self-awareness: If done in a classroom context, did you wait to be chosen or did you choose your partner? What were you feeling when asked to undertake this exercise? How do you feel about working with this other person? And what does the exercise say about you?)

In trying to cement an understanding of empathy it may also be helpful to look at the work of Kunyk and Olson (2001), who identified five ways of understanding empathy, namely as being a human trait: a professional way of being and a form of communication, as well as being a form of communication and a form of relationship. Certainly, empathy has been identified as being vital in forging and maintaining effective therapeutic relationships, which in turn is a vital element of helping others, and generating positive experiences of health and social care (Clark 2010). For example, a clear understanding of the patient's perspective on his or her issues allows not only accurate formulation of the problem but also enables focused intervention, particularly when underpinned by other EI capabilities such as communication.

We might even consider empathy as being purposeful compassion in that through utilising empathic rather than sympathetic communication, we acknowledge the distress of another person and that we are willing to act upon this acknowledgment.

Our actions must be underpinned by ethical codes and ethical reasoning, which in turn require us to have an understanding of the other person's situation. Skoe (2010) and Myrrya (2010) both agree that there is an important relationship between empathy and ethical caring. One such aspect of empathy being central to ethical care is in the consideration of power differentials between the practitioner and the patient.

Empathy is clearly an important capability to have, and yet academic courses within health and social care may not necessarily support the development of EI. You may find your professional training more closely aligned to IQ than to EI. Austin *et al.* (2007) identified that the empathy level of medical students decreased over their training, while Cadman and Brewer (2001), Hurley (2008b) and Freshwater and Stickley (2004) all highlight that professional training often misses out on the enhancement of EI capabilities such as self-awareness and empathy.

Empathy: learning from the field of mental health advocacy

Most of us need to cultivate and develop our EI, and empathy is something that can be cultivated relatively easily in most of us. Empathy is more than just a set of attitudes and beliefs about people, it is a practice, something to work on every day, because it is certainly something that will be challenged in the busy, high-pressure world of work. Indeed, empathy is a verb.

It seems obvious that to cultivate empathy for people who are in distress or suffering, we need to know more about their experience of the world. It also helps to have some awareness of the bigger picture. This understanding promotes empathy to the conditions that promote good health and the links between poverty, violence, disadvantage and poor health outcomes.

There are a disproportionate number of people with mental illness who are incarcerated, and a disproportionate number of homeless people with mental illness, issues which tell us something about both the absence of services and support. It also powerfully illustrates what such absences do to further heighten the vulnerabilities of people with mental illness to unemployment, to losing their homes and livelihood, or to finding themselves on the wrong side of the law. Understanding that the prevalence of mental illness is higher among people who are separated or divorced and lower among those who are married or in long-term relationships might help appreciate how cripplingly lonely the world can be when you're out of step with other people. Part of cultivating empathy, in addition to an appreciation for the bigger picture, is an understanding of what often prevents people from seeking treatment for mental health issues, what forces many to suffer alone – shame. Without stigma, there would be no shame. The effects of stigmatising people with mental illness are far-reaching. The impact of shame and stigma on the individual is rarely considered as part of a general psychiatric assessment, and yet its presence within such assessments may communicate a type of organisational empathy.

While these facts and figures in themselves might not automatically cultivate empathy, reflecting on how this bigger picture impacts on the person sitting in front of you may deepen respect and appreciation for the challenges they may have faced in their lives. Alongside the troubling statistics are the hundreds of positive stories of people who against all the odds have found appropriate treatment and management for mental illness and are living ordinary lives. Campaigns such as 'It's Only 1/100th of Me' (NSW Consumer Advisory Group – Mental Health Inc. 2010) from part of the greater raising on awareness and should be something that nurses and other professionals become familiar with and support.

Cultivating empathy by actively seeking to understanding more about someone else's experience requires all of us to practice listening in an active sense.

We must resist the urge to judge, label or 'know best'. This is particularly salient for those of us who are trained as professionals and are often invited to have the 'answers'. The medical model upon which most of psychiatry is based groups symptoms or behaviours under particular labels, which will be discussed later in this text, and can have devastating impact on the people concerned. The Diagnostic and Statistical Manual of Mental Disorders (DSM) has a seductive kind of certainty; both of these things mean we often find ourselves listening with our own agenda, for boxes to tick, seeing things in one person as 'symptomatic' whereas in someone else not so. Thin clinical definitions of psychosis say nothing of the terror of experiencing a psychotic episode or the courage of surviving it. How hard must it be to try and carry out any everyday activities with such prevalent and relentless negative voices either coming from various sources or just in your own mind.

Cultivating competent practice skills means sitting for sometimes-lengthy periods with lots of contradictions. It helps during these experiences to hold your labels lightly, if you are self-aware enough to know what labels you hold and dispense. If we maintain the view that a diagnosis is not all there is to a person, and practice listening from a 'strengths-based' perspective, we will get a much fuller, richer picture of someone's struggles and his or her life and ultimately what might help. Accepting contradictions and the messiness of all of our lives will guard against putting your own standards, values and belief systems onto others.

Empathy: reflections on a true story

Many years ago I worked in a disability advocacy organisation, during a period when a colleague was having a very hard time. My colleague, Susan, had recently learned her mother had been diagnosed with an aggressive form of ovarian cancer. As a small, close-knit work team, we showed Susan support in the way we knew best. Knowing she was spending all of her free time caring for her mother, we covered the more difficult shifts for her without complaint. We bought her facials and pamper packs. We asked about her mum's progress regularly and listened to the awful details of radiotherapy, hair loss and so on. A few members of the team actually made and home delivered a casserole or two. One Monday morning, Susan stood in the middle of the office and called out to us all:

'Everyone, guys, can you all listen? I know you're all going to ask me, so it's easier I tell you all at once than have to tell you individually. Mum is extremely sick, she's decided she doesn't want to do any more chemo. I'll be off every Friday from now looking after her. Thanks for your support.'

After the update she became teary, and we all rallied around, expressed our sympathies, and empathised as best we could.

During the same time, this writer's father was having one of his periodic bouts of mania. As was his wont, at the first signs of racing thoughts, anxiety and insomnia, he had begun drinking. From his perspective, alcohol slowed down his thinking, took off the edge, and its disinhibiting effect stopped him from worrying about the other things that were happening in his mind. But from everyone else's perspective the booze turned a quiet, sweet, generous man into a grandiose and belligerent pain in the backside. The mania seemed to enhance his physical frailty (he also had diabetes and cirrhosis) to an unbearable degree. He was verbally abusive, mocking and ridiculing anyone who begged to differ, provoked arguments, talked to himself in an excited manner and played Wagner at top volume for hours long into the night. He took to driving along the steep, narrow country lanes near their home, well over the legal limit, and inexplicably one day, he even changed his name. In his mid-70s, underneath the florid side of it all, there was a vulnerability and a deep loneliness about him that made me worry that this bout of 'un-wellness' could be his last.

As usual, my dad refused to see any mental health professionals. When we persuaded a few mental health nurses to come to the house, they immediately started talking about medication, whereupon Dad turned away from them and sat silently, staring at the wall, refusing to answer any questions, so they left. Without the opportunity to spend time with him and get to know him a little they went straight to the option of sedating drugs. When he refused to discuss anything with him, they described him as 'insightless'. Without mental health support, counselling or therapy, the family and my dad did then as had always been done: assumed a sort of 'brace position', hoping that the storm would eventually pass.

No one at work ever knew what was going on. Cancer elicits flowers and well wishes, and every effort to make the sufferer and their carers as comfortable as possible. Empathy flows readily. This is not to suggest that cancer isn't a terrible thing to witness, but it is socially acceptable in a way that mental illness is not. It is rare to have anyone imply directly or indirectly that the cancer sufferer has done something to cause his or her illness. It seems that, as a rule, the more obviously that suffering is linked to some sort of mental health problem, the more there is a tendency for the community to believe that the person in pain has done something to bring this situation upon him- or herself.

Susan's mother's decision to forgo treatment was not judged in the same way the decision to forgo mental health treatment would have been, had our family spoken out about it. Dad's suffering invited assumptions that any resistance to sedatives meant he wasn't 'helping' himself. And we expected to find the same sorts of attitudes elsewhere.

Box 3.7 Reflective activity

- How might empathic work practices challenge key issues from this story?
- What could clinicians and facilities do to reduce this black-and-white thinking about mental health?
- If part of dealing with stigma is challenging stigma, what role could mental health professionals play in this process?

- How might you approach an initial assessment using an understanding of the impact of stigma?
- What sorts of services do you think might be provided if the stigma of mental illness were removed?

CONCLUSION

Practitioners should be encouraged to pursue the twin capabilities of self-awareness and empathy and seek to incorporate them into their clinical practice. This involves being open to self-exploration of the many things that make people what they are; thoughts, needs, emotions, values, defences, actions, communications, problems and goals. Feelings related to these experiences should be focused upon, explored and utilised in supporting and helping others. Viewed in this light it is easy to see why the foremost writers within the filed have incorporated self-awareness and empathy into their models of EI.

REFERENCES

Atwell R, Fulford B. The Christian tradition of spiritual direction as a sketch for a strong theology of diversity. In: Cox J, Campbell A, Fulford B, editors. *Medicine of the Person: faith, science and values in health care provision.* London: Jessica Kingsley Publishers; 2007. pp. 83–95.

Austin E, Evans P, Magnus B, *et al.* A preliminary study of empathy, emotional intelligence and examination performance in MBChB students. *Med Educ.* 2007; **41**(7): 684–9.

Bar-On R, editor. *The Handbook of Emotional Intelligence: the theory and practice of development, evaluation, education and implementation – at home, school and the workplace.* San Francisco, CA: Jossey-Bass; 2000.

Beech BF. The strengths and weaknesses of cognitive behavioural approaches to treating depression and their potential for wider utilization by mental health nurses. *J Psychiatr Ment Health Nurs.* 2000; **7**(4): 343–54.

Ben-Artzi E, Mikulincer M, Glaubman H. The multifaceted nature of self-consciousness: conceptualization, measurement and consequences. *Imagin Cogn Pers.* 1995; **15**(1): 17–43.

Bhugra D. Hindu and Ayurvedic understandings of the person. In: Cox, Campbell, Fulford, op. cit.

Cadman C, Brewer J. Emotional intelligence: a vital ingredient for recruitment in nursing. *J Nurs Manag.* 2001; **9**(6): 321–4.

Campbell J. The relationship of nursing and self-awareness. *Adv Nurs Sci.* 1980; **2**(4): 15–25.

Clark A. Empathy and sympathy: therapeutic distinctions in counselling. *J Ment Health.* 2010; **32**(2): 95–101.

Clarkson P. *Gestalt Counselling in Action.* London: Sage Publications; 1989.

Cox J, Campbell A, Fulford B, editors. *Medicine of the Person: faith, science and values in health care provision.* London: Jessica Kingsley; 2007.

Ehrich L. Phenomenology: the quest for meaning. In: O'Donoghue T, Punch K, editors. *Qualitative Educational Research in Action: doing and reflecting.* London: Routledge Falmer; 2003. pp. 49–60.

Freshwater D, Stickley T. The heart of the art: emotional intelligence in nurse education. *Nursing Inquiry.* 2004; **11**(2): 91–8.

Gardner H. *Multiple Intelligences: the theory in practice.* New York: Basic Books; 1993.

Gardner H. Are there additional intelligences? The case for naturalistic, spiritual and existential intelligences. In: Kane J, editor. *Education, Information and Transformation.* Upper Saddle River, NJ: Prentice Hall; 1999. pp. 111–31.

Gergen K. *An Invitation to Social Construction.* London: Sage Publications; 1999.

Gergen K. *Social Construction in Context.* London: Sage Publications; 2001.

Goleman D. *Emotional Intelligence: why it can matter more than IQ.* 10th ed. New York: Bantam Books; 1995.

Hurley J. Invade your own privacy. *International Journal of Pedagogies and Learning.* 2008; **4**(1): 5–13.

Hurley J. The necessity and barriers for enhancing emotionally intelligent mental health nurses. *Journal of Psychiatric and Mental Health Nursing.* 2008b; **15**(5): 379–85.

Jung CG. The relations between the ego and the unconscious. In: Collected Works of C. G. Jung. Princeton, NJ: Princeton University Press; 1928. pp. 7, 123–241.

Kircher T, David AS. Self-consciousness: an integrative approach from philosophy, psychopathology and the neurosciences. In: Kircher T, David AS, editors. *The Self in Neuroscience and Psychiatry.* Cambridge: Cambridge University Press; 2003.

Kunyk D, Olson JK. Clarification of conceptualizations of empathy. *J Adv Nurs.* 2001; **35**(3): 317–25.

Mayer J, Salovey P. What is emotional intelligence? In: Salovey P, Sluyter D, editors. *Emotional Development and Emotional Intelligence: implications for educators.* New York: Basic Books; 1997. pp. 3–31.

Montgomery C. Coping with the emotional demands of caring. *Adv Pract Nurs Q.* 1997; **3**(1): 76–84.

Morrison T. Emotional intelligence, emotion and social work: context, characteristics, complications and contribution. *Br J Soc Work.* 2007; **37**(2): 245–63.

Myyrya L, Juujärvi S, Pesso K. **Empathy**, perspective taking and personal values as predictors of moral schemas. *J Moral Educ.* 2010; **39**(2): 213–33.

Pawson R, Tilley N. *Realistic Evaluation.* London: Sage; 1997.

Perls F, Hefferline R, Goodman P. *Gestalt Therapy: excitement and growth in the human personality.* New York: Penguin Books; 1973.

Pfeifer H, Cox J. The man and his message. In: Cox J, Campbell A, Fulford B, editors. *Medicine of the Person: faith, science and values in health care provision.* London: Jessica Kingsley Publishers; 2007. pp. 33–45.

Salovey P, Mayer J. Emotional intelligence. *Imagination, Cognition, and Personality.* 1990; **9**(3): 185–211.

Shulman L. *The Skills of Helping: individuals and groups.* Itaska, IL: Peacock Publishers; 1999.

Skoe E. The relationship between empathy-related constructs and care-based moral development in young adulthood. *J Moral Educ.* 2010; **39**(2): 191–211.

Szasz T. The myth of mental illness. In: Szasz T, editor. *Ideology and Insanity: essays on the psychiatric dehumanisation of man.* London: Marion Boyars; 1983. pp. 12–24.

Yontef G. *Awareness, Dialogue, and Process.* Available at: www.gestalt.org/yontef.htm (accessed 17 July 2011).

CHAPTER 4

The therapeutic relationship and emotional intelligence

Paul Linsley and Valeria Carroll

The therapeutic alliance is a collaborative relationship between client and practitioner based on trust and respect. In this relationship the practitioner uses personal attributes and clinical techniques such as emotional intelligence to bring about insight, growth and behavioural change. The process involved in achieving this is complex and requires careful navigation and commitment on part of both the client and practitioner. This chapter examines the different phases of the relationship and highlights the necessary steps and qualities needed to achieve this.

ENGAGEMENT

Engagement has been described as the demonstration of willingness to become involved, the evidence of a desire to pursue an understanding of the patient's situation as they see it (Berg *et al.* 2007). Engagement with the client can be in the form of a one-off conversation, or conversely, a series of meetings. Not all interactions develop into therapeutic relationships but may nonetheless be helpful to the client, for example, in navigating the healthcare system by referral to another more appropriate service. It is through engagement with the client that care and services are developed and new ways of thinking are explored. As with any interaction, practitioners need to be mindful as to the message they convey and seek to ensure that their actions are in keeping with what is expected of them by their profession and more importantly by the client.

Involvement: the key to engagement

Involving the patient in decision-making should be a given within any healthcare system that seeks to promote independence in those that it serves. An interesting notion and one that fits well with the philosophy and underpinnings of EI is the concept of humanisation – the notion of upholding a particular view or value of what it means to be human. The conceptual framework put forward by professors Immy Holloway, Kate Galvin and Les Todres of Bournemouth University (Todres *et al.* 2009) argues that most health and social care practitioners enter their chosen profession with a strong sense of empathy for the human plight. However, this emotional resource is difficult to sustain over time, particularly when subject to a working environment that increasingly promotes technological procedures and a distancing from the patient. The conceptual framework they provide proposes eight dimensions that could be fruitfully attended to when thinking about how we interact and provide services to others. These dimensions are:

- **insiderness**: connecting with people's 'inward sense' of how they are: avoiding interactions and strategies that make people feel excessively like 'objects'
- **agency**: finding ways to enhance peoples' sense of being an active participant in their care: avoiding interactions and strategies that reduce human dignity by emphasising people's passivity
- **uniqueness**: finding ways in which people can feel that they are being seen for themselves and not just how they fit into a category or diagnosis
- **togetherness**: finding ways that can enhance our need for belonging: to find familiar interpersonal connections so that our sense of isolation is reduced when facing various health conditions and treatment regimes
- **sense-making**: finding ways to communicate so that people don't just feel like a 'cog in a wheel', rather than what is being offered makes sense and is fair to them
- **personal journey**: finding ways to help people connect with a sense of historical continuity, 'where they have come from' and 'where they are going'; a sense of personal identity is less likely to be lost when a person's sense of personal story is held onto
- **sense of place**: finding ways to enhance the physical environment around 'care' so that people can feel more 'at home'; avoiding built designs and spaces that do not consider the humanly aesthetic considerations
- **not just a 'body'**: finding ways that help people to expand their horizons and tap into 'well-being' resources that are available beyond just a definition of themselves in terms of their 'illness' or 'symptoms': enhancing all the possible meaningful connections beyond themselves that are possible (Todres *et al.* 2009).

This framework is useful in focusing our interactions with others and challenges the practitioner to think creatively about the ways in which they engage with clients and their families.

THE THERAPEUTIC RELATIONSHIP

The focus of the therapeutic relationship is very much on the client and his or her needs. Attending to a client's needs is a skill in itself and comes with practise and experience. The therapeutic relationship is a complex and dynamic process that involves the practitioner trying to help the client make sense of his emotions and what he is going through. This requires an assessment of events, psychological understanding of the situation, and the planning of goals and alternative ways of coping. The perception cannot be universal in the sense that every patient differs and has different attitudes on various life issues and has varied levels of understanding and withstanding capabilities. To succeed, practitioners must pay attention to their clients in individually and culturally appropriate ways (Sommers-Flanagan and Sommers-Flanagan 2004) – such as intuitive and empathic listening, observing verbal and non-verbal communication, patience, and sensitivity to cultural, spiritual and gender differences. This requires the practitioner to be mindful of the way she responds and reacts to what is being said by the client.

Central to the establishment of the therapeutic relationship is the twin concepts of trust and respect. It is through these that the patient begins to understand that he or she is entering a relationship that is essentially safe, confidential, reliable and consistent with appropriate and clear boundaries (Sommers-Flanagan 2003). In healthcare, a **therapeutic alliance** exists when a client and provider develop a mutual trusting, caring and respectful bond that allows collaboration in care and treatment (King and Wheeler 2006).

This alliance is built over time and is dynamic in nature, and it uses cognitive and affective levels of interaction. Much work is required from both parties in order to develop and maintain this alliance, and it is only through careful monitoring of the relationship by both parties that progress can be measured and disruptions to the therapeutic process identified and addressed. Its nature varies with the context, including physical setting, the kind of service offering the help, the needs of the client, and the experience of the practitioner.

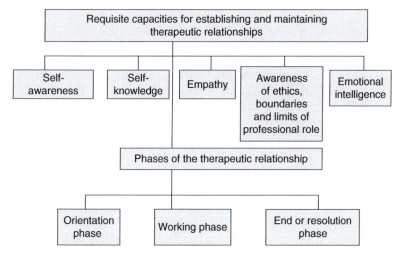

FIGURE 4.1 The therapeutic relationship

The therapeutic relationship can be thought of having three overlapping phases: the orientation phase, the working phase and the end (or resolution) phase. Each phase is characterised by specific client behaviours and goals and different levels of help and input by the practitioner; each represents a way-marker in the client journey and should be celebrated on completion. The relationship does not evolve as a simple, linear relationship. Instead, the relationship may remain predominately in one phase, but reflections of all phases can be seen in each interaction (Forchuck 2000).

Orientation phase

The orientation phase is the first stage of the therapeutic relationship and is really about setting the scene and outlining what is to be expected by both parties with regards to the 'ways of working'. The practitioner and client begin to get to know each other by giving of themselves through disclosure and structured dialogue. It is during such discussions that the purpose, timing and context of the relationship are set and client goals and expectations of the practitioner explored. This stage is especially important because it is the time in which the foundation for the relationship is established. It is during this period of the relationship that trust becomes established or lost. As part of this, the practitioner needs to be clear what he brings to the relationship with regards to experience and skills and must discuss the limitations of what he has to offer. The building of false hope is to be avoided.

It is important to consider this orientation phase from the client's view. This can be an anxious moment for the client as she tries to come to terms with what is being asked of her. Quite often, the person is unclear as to why she has been referred to a particular service or person. This is not necessarily a failing on the part of the referrer but another sign of the anxiety that the person is under, making her forgetful and 'disorientated'. It is up to the practitioner to aid the client in adjusting to her new situation. Appropriate interventions include: reducing the amount of information the client needs to take on board, reducing stimuli wherever possible, and explaining rules and procedures, times, processes, etc.

The most important goal during the orientation phase is to assess the client to determine the client's needs, knowledge base, strengths and limitations, coping mechanisms, and support system. Often clients do not express their needs directly; behaviour is the only clue to their needs. The goal is to determine the real meaning of the behaviour and to assess the client's perception of the most crucial needs and problems.

The reason for seeking help forms the basis of the assessment and is a means of engaging the client. A focus on strengths, coping strategies, hopes and aspirations is essential to recovery and the development of self-management skills. The inclusion of these aspects gives a balanced assessment that recognises potential and capacity for recovery.

Box 4.1   Reflective activity

Reflect on a time when a client first came to you or your mentor for help. Why did he/she do so? Did anything make him/her uncomfortable about asking for help? What did you or the practitioner do to put the client at ease?

Establishing boundaries

A behaviour frequently exhibited by the client during the orientation stage is testing. The client attempts to determine the degree of the practitioner's trustworthiness. Through behaviour, the client asks:

- is this person truly willing to help me?
- is this person competent to help?
- is this person reliable and trustworthy?

Typical 'testing behaviours' might be forgetting about an appointment or arriving late. Clients may also express anger at something the practitioner has to say, or accuse the practitioner of breaking confidentiality. The practitioner answers such questions through consistent, reliable behaviour, which promotes the development of trust.

Practitioners play an active role not only in the treatment and support of patients, but also in setting limits and defining boundaries. The boundaries of the staff–patient relationship are defined by the roles of the staff and patient. It is the staff's responsibility to define the boundaries because, in many instances, circumstances prevent the patient from being able to define them accurately. Professional relationship boundaries are complex and sometimes unclear. Because the patient is asked to share information usually reserved only for intimate relationships, the patient becomes vulnerable and possibly increasingly dependent on staff. The vulnerability and the dependency place the power of the relationship in the hands of the staff. It is the staff member's responsibility to be clear about relationship limits to protect the integrity of the person. If a staff member attempts to meet personal needs through a patient relationship, then professional boundaries are violated. When professional boundaries are violated, the relationship shifts into a non-therapeutic one. In practice, roles cannot easily be compartmentalised, as they have elaborate interconnections with each other. Some of the behaviour demonstrated in the role of a friend may be replicated in the role of the practitioner. Although some of the behaviour expected in one role may be complementary to another, there may be circumstances when roles are in tension; for instance, it might be unwise to reveal things of a personal nature to the patient.

Barriers to the therapeutic relationship

There are different classifications of barriers devoted to communication in the health and social care sector (O' Toole 2008, Wood 2004) – which emphasise either external or internal origins of barriers. For example, Watkins (1990) suggests the following factors that may become barriers in engaging with clients:

- **secret agendas:** not being honest with the client, not putting the client first
- **inflexibility of context:** the practitioner's reluctance to be flexible in where to meet, times, etc.
- **fears of intimacy:** a practitioner's own issues, his or her personal history, feeling vulnerable/inexperienced due to previous contact with clients
- **insensitivity** to race, culture, gender, values, beliefs
- using previous history and **making assumptions** about a client
- **personal beliefs** and **prejudices**
- making sweeping generalisations and judgements about clients and their needs (**practitioner knows best**).

The external barriers appear due to existing social divisions (race/ethnicity, class, religion, gender, etc.) or physical distractions (interruptions, time pressure, noise, etc.) and are evident to the practitioner by their nature. Identification of these barriers is vital to achieve effective therapeutic relationships, and you are required to be flexible in adjusting and adapting the environment to a therapeutic setting for the purpose of engagement with the client. At the same time it is essential to consider the client's views and his/her emotions and feelings regarding existing external barriers, because our individual perception brings the subjectivity, bias in interpretation due to individual semantics, and personal meaning of the specific barrier, e.g. one might have higher tolerance of noise than another; one might feel stronger about his or her gender identity than another. Therefore, equal contribution from the client and the practitioner to the dialogue about barriers might be beneficial to correct identification of barriers and successfully work at aiming to reduce them.

Box 4.2   Activity

Imagine that during the next session with a client you identified at least three types of external barriers (for example, you might wish to consider gender, age and ethnicity barriers). How are you going to reduce the effect of these barriers? Pay attention to the client's perspective as well.

The internal barriers are subjective barriers and therefore require EI to be identified and addressed. These are the barriers that need practitioners' awareness not only on the cognitive level 'I know' ('read about this'; 'heard about this'), but also on the emotional level 'I feel' ('I feel the tension', 'I do not feel for my client'). At this point, EI might be considered as a tool for personal and professional development, because we need to be prepared to accept that this internal barrier exists and we are the bearers of these barriers. Once we have reached this point of self-awareness and accepted the idea that we display the internal barriers, we can analyse the origins of

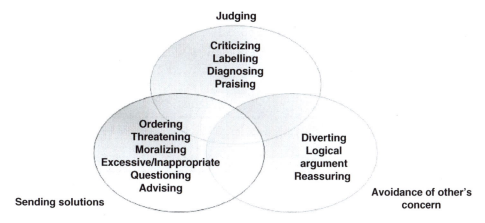

FIGURE 4.2 Internal barriers (Reproduced from J Stewart, *Bridges not Walls: a book about interpersonal communication.* © The McGraw-Hill Companies Inc.)

a particular barrier, its function (Why do we need this barrier? Does it help me to feel better?), and how we can address and reduce this barrier influence.

One of the examples of the internal barriers could be given with the illustration of 'high-risk responses', which Bolton (1995) divided into three categories: judging, sending solutions and avoidance of other's concern (*see* Figure 4.2).

Addressing internal barriers can be achieved if you allow your emotional indicators to support your decisions. Yes, it is important to be able to name different types of barriers; however, for therapeutic purposes it is more essential to feel – if the tension appeared between you and your client – if emotionally you understand your client, or if you feel that there is a block between you both or you do not reach emotionally to your client. To consider the external barriers is only half the way to effective relationships with your client. Focus should be made on internal, emotional factors as well, which very often we underestimate due to their influence on our everyday routine. This leads to established behavioural patterns that we demonstrate during the communication process and that we are used to but might not be successful with a particular individual/client. As the opposite, some might consider particular strategies that have been observed as effective with other clients; however, a more sensitive approach to the individual emotional state of the client and his/her needs could increase emotional bond between practitioner and client, therefore supporting therapeutic outcomes.

Working towards reducing barriers that appear during the therapeutic relationships is often suggested through application of the person-centred approach principles, one of the main principles of which is development of the non-judgemental attitude to the client. However, knowledge of the approach principles does not necessarily lead towards their implementation and can only be achieved if a practitioner is constantly working with his or her emotional component of self. For example, it might be challenging for one not to analyse his client behaviour, as this might be considered to have certain benefits from a practitioner's point of view. However, this barrier increases the already existing power imbalance and therefore further distances practitioners emotionally from their clients. As a result, this might trigger a client's resistance, which leads to vicious circle when actions/reactions of one lead to further resentment of another, and the involvement has emotional direction away from each other rather than towards each other.

Another very common response from a practitioner that blocks emotional engagement with the client is related to 'praising' (Gordon 1970, as cited in Bolton 1995), which many practitioners tend to use as a technique opposite to criticism. This technique is considered in anticipation of positive impact on client's self-esteem and therefore is seen as having some therapeutic value. Particularly, this type of barrier has its popularity due to immediate emotional effect, indicating positive reaction, which can be observed by a practitioner. However, this technique might have the opposite result, impacting therapeutic relationships.

Box 4.3 Reflective activity

From your practice situations, try to recall when you used such adjectives as 'good' or other positive evaluative comments towards your clients (use one for the next activity). You might point out that this technique has been received with 'pleasure' by your client. What was your agenda in using this technique?

Box 4.4 Activity

Based on the recollection of the practice situation with the client, when praise was used, try to imagine the same dialogue, but this time 'your part' is given to a client, who still pays the role of the client. How did you feel being 'praised' by your client?

This activity might have illuminated a certain power imbalance, which distanced you further emotionally further from the client. However, it is important to consider that the interaction with the client, as a two-way process, can be influenced by a client as much as it can be influenced by the professional. You might feel that you are expected to provide positive evaluation in the form of praise, particularly with some individuals who seek your approval. At this point it is important to be aware of the therapeutic purposes of the relationships. It is worth considering that you are responsible for creating opportunities for the client to find his or her own strengths and value of self and therefore to grow and/or remain as an independent individual.

These latter points highlight the importance of being self-aware and emotionally responsive not only to what the client might say or do, but to how the practitioner thinks and conducts him- or herself.

Working phase

During the middle, or *working*, phase of the relationship, the practitioner and the client get to know each other better and test the structure of the relationship to be able to trust one another. Most of the therapeutic work is carried out during the working phase. The practitioner and the client explore relevant stressors and promote the development of insight in the client by linking perceptions, thoughts, feelings and behaviours. These insights should be translated into action and integrated into the person's life experiences. The practitioner is careful to assess correctly the degree of dependency that is necessary for the particular client. Plans may be devised for improved ways of coping with problems and achieving goals. The promotion of problem-solving skills is important in achieving recovery. Old coping skills are not discarded, but instead reviewed as to their appropriateness when dealing with current and past issues. This bolstering of existing skills recognises that the client is not defenseless, and it comes with life experience. Evaluation and redefining of problems also occurs in this phase. The practitioner needs to be alert to the danger of losing objectivity during this time. Any successes, especially instigated and auctioned by the client, should be celebrated.

Jones (1995) identified specific tasks of the working phase of the practitioner–client relationship that are still relevant to current practice:

- maintain the relationship
- gather further data
- promote the client's problem-solving skills, self-esteem and use of language
- facilitate behavioural change
- overcome resistance behaviours
- evaluate problems and goals, and redefine them as necessary
- promote practice and expression of alternative, adaptive behaviours.

Resolution phase

The last phase, resolution, ideally occurs when the goals of the relationship have been accomplished, when both the client and the practitioner feel a sense of resolution and satisfaction. Learning is maximised, and accomplishments are again emphasised and reinforced with the client. Final maintenance of therapeutic parameters occurs; this is to ensure that the client fully understands that the support of the practitioner is at an end. The resolution phase can prove difficult for both client and practitioner. Although agreement between client and practitioner is desirable in deciding when to end the relationship, this is not always possible. Nonetheless, the practitioner's tasks during this phase revolve around establishing the reality of the separation. Stuart (1998) suggests the following criteria for determining client readiness for ending the relationship:

- the patient experiences relief from the presenting problem
- the client's functioning has improved
- the client has increased self-esteem and a stronger sense of identity
- the client uses more adaptive coping responses
- the client has achieved the planned treatment outcomes
- an impasse has been reached in the client–practitioner relationship that cannot be worked through.

EMOTIONAL INTELLIGENCE AS A BASIS FOR THERAPEUTIC INTERVENTION

Emotional intelligence involves the ability to perceive accurately, appraise and express emotion; the ability to access and/or generate feelings when they facilitate thought; the ability to understand emotion and emotional knowledge; and the ability to regulate emotions to promote emotional and intellectual growth (Salovey and Mayer 1997). This emotional mastery is central to the development and maintenance of the therapeutic relationship. It is through a combination of these abilities that the practitioner explores the feelings and thoughts, emotions and behaviour of the client in a structured and helpful manner. In order to do this, the practitioner needs to be aware of his or her own feelings and thoughts and how he or she responds to what is being said by the client. This self-awareness enables the practitioner to guide and support the client in a way that is not only helpful but insightful. It should also be recognised that the practitioners are confronted not only by the client's emotions but also their own. The practitioner must also be aware of prejudicial, conventional, sociocultural norms that are part of their intrinsic moral value system that can be and occluded or ignored (Carveth 2009). These may interfere with and distort the practitioner's perspective of a client, if not safeguarded against. The practitioner attends to these feelings and beliefs in a number of ways: through self-analysis, supervision with a senior clinician, peer supervision or by seeking therapy for themselves.

Emotional intelligence therefore plays an important part in supporting and guiding both the client and practitioner through the phases of the therapeutic relationship. This process can be viewed be viewed in two ways: 1) the practitioner's perception and understanding of the client's emotions, and 2) the practitioner's utilisation of these perceptions to achieve the goal of managing complex situations towards quality patient care. Salovey and Mayer (1997) offer diagrammatical representation of how this process might be utilised for the benefit of both the client and practitioner (*see* Figure 4.3).

Box 4.5   Reflective activity

Reflect on the time you have had with clients. How easy is it to terminate a relationship and say goodbye?

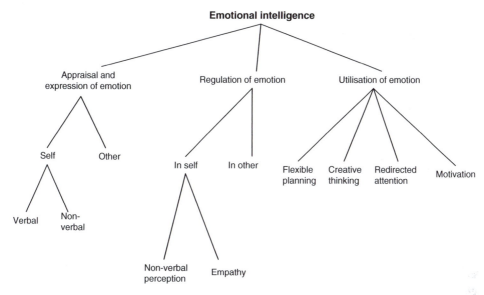

FIGURE 4.3 Emotional intelligence: its role in the therapeutic relationship

The importance of being self-aware and empathic is again highlighted within the model. Also highlighted is the need to be flexible in planning care and creative in how client needs are met and responded to. Using EI in this way can:

- provide the opportunity to discuss and manage emotional states, particularly with regards to stressful or upsetting states
- help to recognise and manage the emotions of others
- provide the basis for intervention and change
- help to deal with conflict situations.

Mayer and Salovey (2000) break the use of EI down even further into four branches of skills. Whilst the Mayer–Salovey Four-Branch Model of EI was developed for leadership and management, with slight adaptation it proves an insightful tool for exploring emotion within the therapeutic relationship. The four branches of the Mayer–Salovey Model and some of their interrelationships are shown in the Figure 4.4.

The first two branches, Perception and Facilitation, are termed 'experiential EI' because they relate most closely to feelings. First, they involve the capacity to perceive emotions in others accurately, and second, the ability to use emotions to enhance how we think. The third and fourth areas of EI skills are termed Strategic EI because they pertain to calculating and planning with information about emotions. The third area, Understanding Emotions, involves knowing how emotions change in and of themselves, as well as how they will change people and their behaviours over time. The fourth area, Emotional Management, focuses on how to integrate

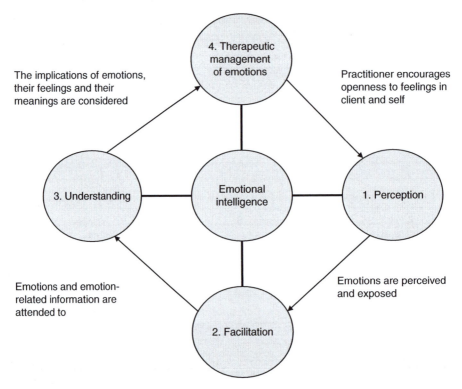

FIGURE 4.4 The Mayer–Salovey Four-Branch Model of EI

logic and emotion for effective decision-making and planning. These four skill areas are related to one another, but they are functionally distinct as well.

> **Box 4.6**   Reflective activity
>
> Reflect on the way in which you currently handle emotion as part of your clinical practice. Are there areas for improvement?

THERAPEUTIC OUTCOMES

The therapeutic relationship is purposeful in that it seeks to support the client through care and treatment aimed at specific desired outcomes, usually that of independent living.

The work of Imogene King emerged in the 1960s and centred upon the interpersonal communications between individuals. King's theory was tightly bound to nursing, but since the first publications of the theory it has held an important position in social care, advocacy, mental nursing, probation services and even management and marketing, and is the foundation of much contemporary thinking on communication within caring contexts. Hence it remains a seminal reference point for assessing and exploring client needs, as well as the setting of therapeutic outcomes (Burnard and Gill 2009, Stein-Parbury 2009).

King identified that a person's goal attainment comprised of three interlocking factors:

- the personal (self)
- the interpersonal (communication and interaction with specific individuals)
- the social systems (self and society).

The personal and social systems factors have an influence on standards and quality of care, but it is the interpersonal factor that leads directly to the success (or otherwise) of goal or outcome attainment. The personal factor includes every aspect of the individual's life and needs. It encompasses a past and a present. Therefore it allows for the individual to have a value above the assessed needs. Within this aspect it is possible to make comparisons of need against status and class. It also incorporates an element of expectation and a reality of situation for the individual. For example, the labourer will aspire to ambitions within the realms of success appropriate to the status of a labourer. A financial windfall will not broaden the outlook, but might improve the material surroundings. On the other hand, the aristocrat will probably have a focus that does not include ambition in the way that the labourer would have. A financial windfall might be of interest, but is likely to be handled differently. The material surroundings of the aristocrat would be of a high standard in the first place.

The two examples also accept that the individual has a unique identity. A significant part of identity is value of the self. Hence a person who is contemplating suicide might say that he or she is worthless (a social value) and can't see any alternative to suicide (an appraisal of personal value and lack of a future context). In this example, the practitioner (interpersonal) brings a new dynamic to the state of understanding. The person contemplating suicide might accept that a practitioner is appropriate in what he or she has to say and suggest and might listen. At some point it might be evident that the practitioner shows an understanding for the plight of the individual (empathy and interaction) and might suggest a simple course of action (involvement of emotion, which is a component of empathy).

Most importantly, the interpersonal interaction allows for a future context to be reiterated. This is significant in that it explicitly allows for hope, change, improvement and newness to be involved in the process of living. The suicidal client meets with denial on the concept of future, and particularly on the concept of a positive and better future. Interpersonal interactions reinforce the positive notion of future in subtle ways. For example, when the person understands that an appointment with a practitioner is imminent, or that an event that might be considered positive is imminent, a degree of hope enters the situation and the expectation of the meeting is an expectation of a future, albeit a short-term future. It is by building upon such short terms that hope and eventually a new purpose can be assured.

The model of King's theory is described by the PIESS mnemonic:

Physical: two concepts of growth and development link and stand as a continuum. There is a known history of growth in that the individual can understand the progress he or she has made in physical growth from childhood to adulthood. Likewise, there is a known history of development in that the same history includes the development of interests, fashions, trends and where an institutional background is involved, staff turnover. Thus time becomes an important part of the physical aspects of life. Time is another continuum that began in the distant past and has moved to the present. It offers a notion of future.

Intellectual: The use of the past by the recollection of events that occurred. The assessment of the recollections will give an indication of the current mood environment. For example, a propensity for recalling happy days will indicate a contented disposition. Conversely, the regular recollections of frustrations, regretful incidents and negative conversations will indicate a negative disposition. The assessor must be alert to acknowledge that the seemingly continuous negativity of the conversation might be due entirely to the person being very uncomfortable or disappointed, or unhappy with the present situation. It might be that if the present situation is improved, then the memories and recollections will be positive.

Emotional: The achievement of self-satisfaction. The individuals who are involved in the interpersonal transactions share information and the person makes the choice to do something to contribute to the required improvement in his or her situation. In this way the emotional involvement is necessarily narcissistic and egocentric. By appealing to the self this way the value of the process of whatever the situation demands is underpinned by the determination to achieve a prescribed outcome. All human emotion is either positively or negatively predisposed towards the enhancement of gratification and pleasure of the individual.

Social: to indulge appropriately in social function. To be involved in the community as an individual who belongs to a group, which in turn is a component of the community. Value is placed on one's position in society. Much of the social value depends upon material wealth and the ability to be self-supporting. This is true of all cultures in every society across the world. The dependency upon others for one's everyday needs and the inability to provide even the basic needs for one's self lead directly to negative moods. This is particularly strong in some patriarchal societies and where the male is dominant.

Western societies have an infrastructure of care that supports disabled and mentally ill people. Legislation provides local authorities with a duty to provide care appropriate to need. The social factors also include the need to establish meaningful relationships with other individuals. A society exists partly because individuals want to communicate with each other. Relationships take different forms. A professional relationship is not the same as a domestic relationship. There are many types and styles of relationships between these two examples. Each individual will seek to experience different relationships across the continuum.

<u>Spiritual</u>: how the individual addresses self-worth in the context of stresses such as personal, interpersonal and social growth: the individual's relationship within his or her own self; the personal value one has and how the individual assesses personal growth. The spiritual person is concerned with purpose. A belief that life includes a dimension of spirituality is only one factor. Religion provides a pathway for development for some people. Others might consider religion to be less or more important than that. The core of the spiritual factor is its subjectivity and the experience of self. This is the inner centre of the individual where ultimately the decision is made about life, death and the value of the personal self.

Box 4.7   Clinical activity

Pay attention to how different practitioners work with clients in assessing for and negotiating therapeutic outcomes. To what extent is emotional intelligence used in the setting of therapeutic outcomes?

Another useful model that may serve as a helpful reference point when exploring the needs of clients and setting therapeutic outcomes is the Five Areas Cognitive Model (Williams 2001).

The **'five areas'** are:

- **altered thinking** – reduction in self-esteem and self-confidence
- **altered feelings (mood and emotions)** – feelings of depression, loss of interest in things and loss of enjoyment
- **physical feelings and symptoms in the body** – altered sleep pattern, fatigue, loss of libido, poor concentration, appetite changes and loss of energy
- **altered behaviour** – change in social or work activity and/or family relationships
- **altered life situation** – practical difficulties and problems, such as finance, home maintenance, etc.

This straightforward assessment is a useful tool for discussing and setting client goals and is one used by the authors.

CONCLUSION

Whatever approach is used in assessing for and setting therapeutic goals, practitioners need to be resourceful and draw on a variety of psychological skills and interventions to facilitate the care and treatment of individual patients and their families, in hospital and community settings. EI provides a means by which to navigate the therapeutic process and plan and structure care. The therapeutic relationship takes time to establish and relies on the participation of the client in making it a meaningful and purposeful exchange.

REFERENCES

Berg WK, Wacker DP, Cigrand K, *et al.* Comparing functional analysis and paired-choice assessment results in classroom settings. *J Appl Behav Anal.* 2007; **40**(3): 545–52.

Bolton R. Barriers to communication: common communication spoilers. In: Stewart J, editor. *Bridges, not Walls: a book about interpersonal communication.* 6th ed. New York: McGraw-Hill; 1995. pp. 134–45.

Burnard P, Gill P. *Culture, Communication and Nursing.* Harlow: Pearson Education; 2009.

Campbell J. The relationship of nursing and self-awareness. *Adv Nurs Sci.* 1980; **2**(4): 15–25.

Carveth D. *What Does Psychoanalysis Have to Learn from Existentialism?* [Unpublished paper]. Paper presented at: Toronto Psychoanalytic Society; 11 February 2009.

Forchuck C, Westwell J, Martin ML, *et al.* The developing nurse-client relationship: nurses' perspectives. *J Am Psychiatr Nurses Assoc.* 2000; **6**(1): 3–10.

Jones A. The organisational influence on counseling relationships in a general hospital setting. *J Psychiatr Ment Health Nurs.* 1995; **2**(2): 83–5.

King D, Wheeler S. *Supervising Counsellors: issues of responsibility.* London: Sage; 2009.

Mayer JD, Salovey P, Caruso D. Models of emotional intelligence. In: Sternberg RJ, editor. *The Handbook of Intelligence.* New York: Cambridge University Press; (2000). pp. 396–420.

O'Toole G. *Communication: Ccore interpersonal skills for health professionals.* Sydney: Elsevier; 2008.

Salovey P, Mayer JD. What is emotional intelligence? In: Salovey P, Sluyter D, editors. *Emotional Development and Emotional Intelligence: implications for educators.* New York: Basic Books; 1997. pp. 3–31.

Sommers-Flanagan J, Sommers-Flanagan, R. *Clinical interviewing.* 3rd ed. Hoboken, NJ: Wiley; 2003.

Sommers-Flanagan J, Sommers-Flanagan R. *Counselling and Psychotherapy Theories in Context and Practice.* London: Wiley; 2004.

Stein-Parbury J. *Patient and Person: interpersonal skills in nursing.* 4th ed. Marrickville: Elsevier Churchill Livingstone; 2009.

Stuart GW. Therapeutic nurse-patient relationship. In: Stuart GW, Laraia MT, editors. *Principles and Practice of Psychiatric Nursing.* 6th ed. New York: Mosby; 1998.

Todres L, Galvin KT, Holloway I. The humanisation of healthcare: a value framework for qualitative research. *Int J Qual Stud Health Well-Being.* 2009; **4**(2): 68–77.

Watkins P. *Communication Skills.* London: New Harbinger Publications; 1990.

Williams C. *Overcoming Depression: a five areas approach.* London: Arnold; 2001.

Wood JT. *Interpersonal Communication: everyday encounters.* Wadsworth/Thomson Learning; 2002.

CHAPTER 5

Communication

Paul Linsley

Good communication is the foundation on which clinical practice is based. As healthcare professionals go about their work they are required to communicate with a number of different people; requiring them to balance conflicting aims, interests, rights and reactions of others with their own agenda. Good communication provides the means by which to manage and deal with these demands, ensuring that the needs of people are not lost in the often confusing world of healthcare. It is a complex process of interaction and exchange between two or more people, requiring attention and thought. In this sense, good communication could be argued an essential skill in being personally effective.

Communication can be defined as the process whereby speech, signs or actions transmit information from one person to another. However, it is much more than this, as Anderson (1959) observed, 'communication is the process by which we understand others and in turn endeavour to be understood by them. It is dynamic, constantly changing and shifting in response to the total situation'. For communication to be effective it needs to be structured in a way that is understood by all those involved and reflective of the circumstances in which it is conducted. In this way, communication is much more than the spoken word but is contained in everything that we say (or don't say) and do (or don't do).

There are mainly three types of communication skills: expressive skills, listening skills and skills for managing the overall process of communication (Hargie and Dickinson 2004). Expressive skills are required to convey a message to others through words, facial expressions and body language. Listening skills are skills that are used to obtain messages or information from others. These help to clearly understand what a person feels and thinks about you or understand the other person closely. Skills for managing the overall process of communication help to recognise the required information and develop a strong hold on the existing rules of communication and interaction. These include how we position ourselves when speaking to another, appearance and professional courtesy, as well as when to interrupt another and move the conversation on. Perhaps the greatest skill, however, is conveying to another that what they have had to say has been acknowledged and understood. There is nothing more frustrating and upsetting than believing that you have not been heard and taken seriously.

THE COMMUNICATION PROCESS

Communication is a complex process which requires careful attention and monitoring. Whilst there are a number of models depicting the communication process, perhaps the best known of these is the structural model of communication (Boyd 1995, p. 431), replicated here (*see* Figure 5.1).

The process involves a sender, a message and a receiver. The sender is the originator of the message. However, in order to do this, the sender needs to formulate an idea of what he or she wants to say, put this into words, and transmit the message with emotion. The receiver then decodes the message (interprets the message

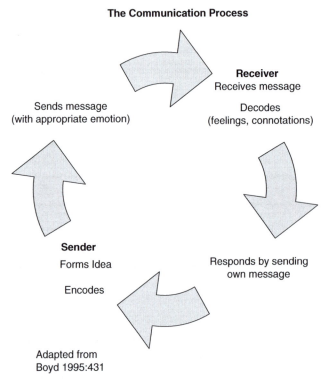

Figure 5.1 Structural model of communication

including its feelings, connotation and context) and then responds, either verbally or by action. The context refers to the setting in which the communication takes place. This is much more than the physical setting, but includes the relationship between the sender and the receiver, their shared understanding of each other, and cultural values and norms, amongst other things. You only communicate when the message you send out has been received, acknowledged and sent back to you, so that you know that it has been properly understood. Communication is ended once either party disengages from this process.

In itself, the process would seem to be quite straightforward; however, there are a number of things that can interfere and get in the way of the message being sent or received (Trevithick *et al.* 2004). If the sender is communicating the same message in what he or she says and does, then this is congruent. However, if the sender says one thing but his gestures and body shape say another, then the communication is incongruent; for example, the person who says that he is happy, with slumped shoulders and downturned mouth. Incongruent messages produce a dilemma for the receiver, who does not know how to respond. Inappropriate messages may cause confusion and distress within the client. Failures in timing, stereotyping the receiver, or not including important information may mean that the essence of what is being said is lost. Another common mistake people make is to focus on the delivery of the information, rather than how it is received. The receiver may miss important verbal and non-verbal clues and misinterpret the intentions and needs of the sender; for example, is the message the practitioner received consistent with the original idea of the client? Did the practitioner interpret the message as the client intended? Focusing on the client and what she has to say, the way in which she says it, and responding appropriately, increases the chances of capturing the message.

Verbal communication

Effective verbal and non-verbal communication skills are a requirement of most jobs, but are highlighted within healthcare as being essential. Communication takes place on two levels: verbal and non-verbal (Hargie 2006). Verbal communication is communication that uses words, either written or spoken. Taken alone, verbal communication can convey factual information accurately and effectively. However, verbal communication is less able to capture and express feelings or nuances of meanings. In this sense verbal communication can be said to contain subjective meaning, which is meaning to the person who spoke or wrote the words. Words seldom mean precisely the same thing to two people. When we say we are 'sad', 'in pain', 'finding it hard going', there is often then a need to clarify these terms in a way that others can understand. This situation can become more complicated as words can change meaning with different cultures and communities. The characteristics of the speaker and the context in which things are said will influence how words and phrases are received and the level to which they are understood. Practitioners should strive to overcome such obstacles by checking their interpretation and incorporating information from the non-verbal level as well.

Non-verbal communication

Non-verbal communication involves everything except the spoken or written word. Non-verbal communication, its interpretation and use, is as important as verbal communication, if not more so in conveying feelings and emotion (McKay, Davis and Fanning 2009). This is because non-verbal communication is often unconsciously motivated and more accurately indicates a person's meaning than the spoken word. So much information can be gleaned from what the person has to say and how they say it. By assessing and paying attention to the person's posture, facial expression and the way that they hold and conduct him- or herself offers insight into the person's character and the way the person feels about a situation or event, as well as their coping strategies. Non-verbal communication cues play a number of roles when transmitting and receiving a message, some of which are listed below (Griffin 1997):

- **repetition:** repeating and emphasising the message the person is making verbally; it helps to maintain the flow of communication and acts as a subtle indicator to show when a person has finished speaking and awaiting a response
- **complementation:** adding to or complementing a verbal message, e.g. a practitioner shaking the hand of a client whilst welcoming him or her can increase the message that the professional is there to help
- **substitution:** adding to or complementing a verbal message; for example, putting a hand round someone's shoulder can reinforce the message that the person is there to support and help the other
- **accenting:** accenting or underlining a verbal message; pounding the table, for example, can underline a message.

Non-verbal communication can distort verbal information as well as enhance it. Lack of facial expression or a monotonous voice, for instance, may act as a barrier to communication. Some non-verbal communication cannot be changed: for example, age, race, sex and physical appearance. A person's accent is another relatively stable characteristic by which people are often evaluated. There is a tendency to make global inferences about people on the basis of very limited information, and to minimise just how much people's behaviour is affected by the situation and environment they are in, especially if they perceive it as strange or intimidating.

Not only is it important to be sensitive to the person's non-verbal communication, but sensitivity to and awareness of our own body signals is also vital. Using body language appropriately in a helping relationship can help to facilitate a client's trust and confidence in the healthcare worker. Tone of voice, eye contact, touch, facial expression and posture can all convey qualities of genuineness and warmth.

Using non-verbal communication effectively can help relax clients to the point that they disclose things that they would not otherwise have done so. In turn, the more relaxed patients feel, the more likely they are to exhibit their usual behaviour.

Practitioners may influence what patients say and how they behave, not only by what they say, but also by their non-verbal communication and use of silence. If healthcare workers only respond positively when patients mention improvement of symptoms, for example, patients may become inhibited about admitting that the condition is static or worsening.

Even when we are silent we still communicate a lot of information to others – through our eyes, facial expression, posture, gestures and personal appearance. Through these non-verbal behaviours we communicate who we are and how we feel. Others draw conclusions about our sincerity, credibility and emotional state based on our non-verbal behaviour. Poor eye contact, slouching, nervous gestures and other non-assertive behaviours can convince others that what we have to say can be safely ignored.

The importance of active listening

The way in which we listen (or fail to listen) can be a major barrier in our inter-personal relationships. It is easy to take listening for granted and, through our own preconceptions, to fail to listen (Freshwater and Stickley 2006, p. 14). If we are to fully understand, we need to learn to listen effectively. We need to listen not only to words, but also to the hidden feelings and intentions that are expressed. This means listening to what a person is saying and making sure the reasons for the consultation are clear. Verbal and non-verbal clues are important and may be missed if full attention is not given to the patient.

Active listening focuses on what the patient is saying, to be able to respond to the message in an objective manner. While listening, the practitioner concentrates only on what the patient is saying and the underlying meaning; this is termed active listening. The practitioner usually responds indirectly using techniques such as open-ended statements, reflection, and questions that elicit additional responses from the patient. In active listening, the practitioner should avoid changing the subject, and instead follow the lead of the patient. However, at times it is necessary to respond directly by using techniques such as questions to help a patient focus on a specific topic. As we listen, we attempt to make sense of, retain and judge what the speaker is saying. We plan what we are going to say in response, and we covertly rehearse our response. There are a number of verbal skills that the practitioner can use to show that they are listening to the client, some of which are listed here (McCabe and Timmins 2006):

- **encouraging:** 'I would like to hear more about how you managed the situation. Could you explain that a little more fully? It's important that we explore that in more depth'
- **acknowledging:** 'I understand', 'I see', 'that sounds really important to you'

- **checking:** 'It appears to me that you are upset by events'
- **clarifying:** 'I'm not sure that I understand. Could you please go over that again?'
- **affirming:** 'I appreciate your honesty and for discussing the matter with me'
- **empathy:** 'I can understand why you behaved the way you did, given the same situation I may well have acted the same way'
- **asking open-ended questions:** 'Can you tell me more about that?'
- **reflecting:** 'You appear to be happy with what was said'
- **summarising:** 'So there seem to be several things that are important to you that you need to remember to mention to the doctor the next time you see him. Would you like me to record them in your notes?'
- **silence:** remaining quiet, but non-verbally expressing interest in what the person is saying through the use of non-verbal cues and prompts.

There are a number of things that can act as a block to listening. These can be overcome with experience and practice, however. Some of the more common mistakes to listening are listed below (Rothwell 2010):

- **comparing:** 'What's he complaining about? There are a lot more patients worse off than him', 'I personally wouldn't have done it that way'; this stops the practitioner hearing what the person has to say and does not recognise the individual's right to make and learn from his or her mistakes
- **mind reading:** trying to figure out what the other person is thinking and feeling; in this way, the listener portrays a sense of mistrust in what the other is saying, paying more attention to subtle changes in intonation and expression rather than the actual words
- **rehearsing:** giving attention to the preparation and delivery of your next comment – this can be the result of inexperience as the new practitioner seeks to say and do the right thing. Some people rehearse whole chains of responses: I'll say, then he'll say, and so on
- **filtering:** listening to some things and not to others – more commonly known as 'selective hearing': hearing what you want to hear and not the rest
- **judging:** not listening to what the person has to say, as you have already judged him
- **advising:** the practitioner feels the need to offer advice; again, this is often a sign of inexperience and a desire to do right by the client – the practitioner hears a few sentences and starts to look for solutions to the client's problem rather than paying attention to the rest of what the client is saying
- **being right:** going to any lengths to avoid being wrong: 'doctor knows best', having the last word
- **dreaming:** half-listening while something the other person says triggers off a chain of associations of your own
- **identifying:** referring everything the other person says to one's own experience
- **advising:** being the great problem solver; offering advice where it is not wanted

- **sparring:** arguing and debating; you disagree so quickly that the other person never feels heard; you take strong stands and are clear about your beliefs, values and preferences
- **derailing:** changing the subject suddenly; for example, making a joke in order to avoid the discomfort or anxiety you might feel if you really listened to the other person
- **placating:** agreeing with everything and not really listening to what is being said – again, this can be a sign of inexperience and a wanting to do right by the client, agreeing eagerly from a desire to please or to seem supportive: 'Right ... absolutely ... I know ... of course you're upset, who wouldn't be?'

Box 5.1 Listening skills

Reflect on the way that you listen or don't listen when engaging with clients. Are there points that you could improve upon? Make a list of these and work to address them.

ENGAGING ANOTHER IN EFFECTIVE COMMUNICATION

In order to engage and connect with another, certain core conditions need to be met and acted upon. These dimensions include genuineness, respect, empathetic understanding and concreteness (Rodgers 1994). It is through these dimensions that the practitioner begins to understand and support the person and by which trust and open communication is fostered. More importantly, the person himself is subject to change through self-understanding and insight.

GENUINENESS

Genuineness requires the practitioner to be open and honest in his or her communication despite what the practitioner may feel about the other person. It is the quality of being authentic; that is, not thinking and feeling one thing and saying and doing something different. Professional conduct requires 'not only expertise and diligence, but honesty and integrity' (Burns and Grove 2005, p. 176). It is through the latter that genuineness is demonstrated and conveyed and by which our behaviour and conduct is measured. Being genuine also implies the ability to use communication tools in a way that is spontaneous and in keeping with self and the context in which the exchange is taking place.

RESPECT

As healthcare professionals we would like to believe that we treat each and every person the same, no matter what the person's circumstances, but as Rose (2004) highlights, 'our views and beliefs can and are challenged in clinical practice when faced with the complexities of human nature'. Probably the hardest thing to do is to respect and support other people for making their own choices, even when you disagree with them. Communication of this kind is about engaging in open and honest debate with the goal of enriching each others' perspectives, not for the purpose of proving someone wrong. Respect is about achieving a high level of functioning within a role, doing the best that we can for the client, and being consistent in what we say and do.

EMPATHETIC UNDERSTANDING

Empathy has been defined by Kalisch (1973) as 'the ability to enter into the life of another person, to accurately perceive his current feelings and their meanings'. Additionally, Rogers (1961) described empathy as 'sensing accurately the feelings and personal meanings the client is experiencing and communicating this acceptant understanding to the client'. Whatever definition is used, empathy signifies a central focus and feeling with and in the client's world and involves the following (Mercer and Reynolds 2002):

- accurately perceiving the client's situation, perspective, and feelings
- communicating one's understanding to the client and checking with the client for accuracy
- acting on this understanding in a helpful way toward the client.

Appropriate use of empathy as a communication tool facilitates the clinical interview, increases the efficiency of gathering information, and puts the client at the centre of what we do. Platt and Keller (1994) provides a number of steps to providing an empathetic response, in which the use of EI could enhance further.

These include recognising the presence of strong feelings; giving thought to how others might be feeling; allowing the exploration and expression of these emotions; and supporting the person in this process.

Empathic understanding also includes the ability to communicate and reflect these feelings back to the client in a constructive way that the client can understand and work with. The real dilemma for the practitioner when using empathic communication comes when finding a middle path between two mistakes: being oblivious to others' feelings and conversely intruding on others' feelings. This is why it is important to let the client lead on such matters, allowing him to disclose and feel safe in the expression of his emotions, whilst recognising and conveying what it is he is going through and how he is feeling and responding that situation.

CONCRETENESS

Concreteness means being specific and factual in what we have to say, avoiding the unnecessary and complicated. Communication should be pitched at the level of the client and is effective when it is understood. Being concise and avoiding jargon are good examples of achieving this.

TRUST

To feel safe in expressing emotional problems and needs, the client must trust that the practitioner will safeguard that information and use it in his or her best interest and not break confidentiality. Effective communication is more than just talking; within the healthcare setting, it is essential for the well-being of those that you care for. In developing trust we call on the qualities already described above, those of genuineness, empathy and respect (both self-respect and respect for the client). In communication, self-respect is achieved by observing personal limits and working within these, being assertive, and clearly communicating expectations.

SELF-AWARENESS

A central concept to the development of EI is to build on personal competence and resilience through the use of self-awareness (*see* Chapter 3, Self-awareness and empathy: foundational skills for practitioners). Self-awareness refers to the recognition of personal strengths and weaknesses in an individual and results in the construction of a picture of how the person is doing within a given context, whether in one's personal or professional life. In order to be worth and to promote development over time, this process should be ongoing and based on a realistic and truthful appraisal of the individual and his or her abilities.

The same holds true for the development and use of effective communication skills (Shattell, Starr and Thomas 2007). As with any skill, communication can be taught and improved with use. Self-awareness allows us to recognise when we do things well and highlights areas for improvement. Effective communication is not only constructed by the process of interaction with others, but with time and experience. A person with a developed sense of self-awareness is not only mindful of how their behaviour and actions are supporting and safeguarding others, but is able to take advantage of opportunities as they present within conversation and guide the communication in a meaningful and constructive way. Being self-aware within communication allows the person to understand how one gathers information, makes decisions, generates energy and voices preferences to others.

A FRAMEWORK OF COMMUNICATION

A complementary framework of communication with which to think about our use of EI in clinical practice is that offered by Hamilton and Martin (2007). In trying to 'capture and complement the varied, eclectic, multi-dimensional and challenging role' of practitioners, the authors sought to develop a framework of communication that offered 'flexibility and versatility', which they asserted are 'the essential qualities of … an effective communicator'.

Box 5.2 A framework for effective communication skills practice (the five 'I's)

1   INTERACT with the patient.

2   Establish the INTENTION of the interaction.

3   Decide on the INTERVENTION to be used.

4   Assess the IMPACT of the intervention/s.

5   Evaluate the IMPLICATIONS of the subsequent information obtained and act accordingly.

(Hamilton and Martin 2007, reproduced with permission of *Nursing Times*)

Interaction

During the course of their work, healthcare practitioners interact with a number of different people from different backgrounds and social standings. This can prove challenging and indeed difficult at times. It requires self-control and discipline, as the practitioner seeks to keep disruptive emotions and impulses under control, and safeguard against these interfering with the care that he or she provides. It also requires constant self-monitoring not only of the self, but the way in which the other person is responding to what is being said and asked of him. Practitioners should employ as full a range of communication skills as is possible to ensure that nothing of importance is lost and instead is highlighted and explored within the interaction. This places a duty on healthcare professionals to ensure that their communication skills are at least sufficient to meet the demands of their profession and those that they care for and support. This also places a duty on the practitioner to be transparent in her assessment of self and her communication with others and to take responsibility for and make good any shortfall in her clinical practice.

It also stresses the importance of the need to safeguard and set internal standards and use initiative, recognising and responding to opportunities as they present. Important here is to allow the patient the time in which to express himself and any concerns that he may have, as well as to explore any options that are available to him. Likewise, the practitioner not only needs to listen to what the patient has to say but the way in which it is said.

Intention

Practitioners should establish their intentions when engaging with others in their care. This encourages the practitioner to think about what it is they are doing and provides a focus for the communication process, and something that can be built upon. This is particularly important, given the pressures of time within the modern healthcare setting. If the practitioner's intent is to break 'bad news', then allowing a short period of time in which to do this is inappropriate and potentially damaging for all those involved. Underlying intentions are those that serve and inform our practice regardless of the purpose of the intervention. Using EI demands that we seek to manage our emotions and safeguard the well-being of the client in whatever we do and undertake.

Interventions to be used

Practitioners also need to decide on the most appropriate interventions to be used. These interventions may take physical or psychological form, depending on the overall aim and purpose of the interaction, for example: administering an injection, carrying out physical observations, assisting the elderly with their activities of daily living, or reassuring an anxious patient using communication skills.

Impact

Practitioners should then proceed to assess the impact of the selected intervention. Has the practitioner achieved what he or she has set out to achieve? If not, why not? What could be done differently next time? These are questions that can be asked during the course of the intervention as well as at the end. Being able to recognise and control feelings is a complex matter and requires thought and attention. Likewise, there is the need to be flexible within communication in order to respond to a person's needs. Staff may feel pressured in what they are doing and respond quickly to a situation without thinking about the consequences or the impact of their actions.

Evaluation

The final step is to evaluate the implications of the interaction for the practitioner and client alike. For example, acquiring new information from a client during an interview may necessitate a change in care. This is turn will need to be communicated and actioned as appropriate to other members of the team and, more importantly, the client.

THE RECOVERY JOURNEY

Modern-day healthcare encourages practitioners to focus on the needs of individuals and to assist them in their journey of recovery. The idea of recovery as a journey is not a new one and has been promoted within mental health for some time now (Barker and Buchanan-Barker 2008), and it:

- provides a holistic view of mental illness that focuses on the person, not just one's symptoms
- believes recovery from severe mental illness is possible
- is a journey rather than a destination
- does not necessarily mean getting back to where the person was before
- happens in 'fits and starts' and, like life, has many ups and downs
- calls for optimism and commitment from all concerned
- is profoundly influenced by people's expectations and attitudes
- requires a well-organised system of support from family, friends or professionals
- requires services to embrace new and innovative ways of working (Buchanan-Barker and Barker 2006).

Whilst the concept was developed in mental health, its principles are applicable to all areas of healthcare. There are a number of definitions of recovery, but the guiding principle is that of hope – the belief that it is possible for someone to regain a meaningful life, despite their illness. As can be imagined, this journey is often a traumatic and emotional one and can contain a number of setbacks. Traditional professional relationships, built on status and hierarchy, may not always support recovery but instead disempower the client by taking away responsibility.

Recovery relationships are built on:

- **empowerment and self-management:** what works for the client rather than what works for the service
- **the 'whole person' approach:** focus on the client and not treatment; strengths rather than weakness; what the client can do, rather than what they can't
- **willingness to go the extra mile** in support of the client.

There can be little doubt that the use of EI leads to more positive attitudes, greater adaptability, improved relationships and increased orientation towards positive values (Kristin and Elisabeth 2007), such as those listed above, and has the potential to assist the client in the process of recovery. The idea within the relationship is not to win the client over to the practitioner's way of thinking but to offer him or her a full and open opportunity to explore the situation and to define the changes that the client wants to make. For example, clients and their families are often asked to provide details about past medical treatments, medication, hospitalisations, and therapies. What is overlooked is the experience of the health problem or the experience of interactions with professionals. Inviting patients and their families to talk about their previous experiences with the healthcare system may highlight their concerns and resources, wishes and needs. The skills of active listening and collaborative communication

> **Box 5.3** A comparison of Traditional and Collaborative Practitioner Communication
>
> *Traditional practitioner communication*
> - One view; that of the service or profession
> - Instruction; practitioner knows best
> - Telling
> - An obscuring of difference
> - Closing down options
>
> *Collaborative communication*
> - Many views; that of the client, practitioner, significant others, etc.
> - Negotiation
> - Sharing
> - Difference
> - Opening up options

(*see* Box 5.3) are vital to this process, as is the management and use of emotion in supporting the client.

The practitioner is not a passive partner in the relationship, but acts as a foil – checking out, sometimes gently challenging ambiguity, but never superimposing her own or her profession's agenda unless there is a real or legal need to do so, i.e. the serious risk of harm. This 'handing over' of responsibility can be a powerful experience in itself. Not everybody is happy taking responsibility for their own well-being, and this can prove to be a difficult time for client and practitioner alike. Discussion of beliefs that prevent the person from taking on responsibility and seeking alternative ways of handling the situation may help the client to take charge of the situation.

CONCLUSION

Good communication skills are fundamental to the practice of healthcare workers, regardless of role. Communication skills are something that can be learned and developed over time. The need to be structured in our communication is highlighted, as is the ability to be flexible in our undertakings. Communication should be purposeful and centred on the client. This requires the practitioner to be self-aware and responsive not only to the emotional well-being of others but also to themselves.

REFERENCES

Anderson M. What is communication? *J Comm.* 1959; 9(5).

Barker P, Buchanan-Barker P. Reclaiming nursing: making it personal. *Mental Health Practice.* 2008; **11**(9): 12–16.

Boyd M. Communication with patients, families, healthcare providers, and diverse cultures. In: Strader M, Decker P, editors. *Role Transition to Patient Care Management.* Norfolk, CT: Appleton & Lange; 1995.

Buchanan-Barker P, Barker P. The ten commitments: a value base for mental health recovery. *Journal of Psychosocial Nursing.* 2006; **44**(9): 29–33.

Burns N, Grove SK. *The Practice of Nursing Research: conduct, critique, and utilization.* 5th ed. St. Louis, MO: Elsevier; 2005.

Freshwater D, Stickley TJ. The heart of the art: emotional intelligence in nurse education. *Nursing Inquiry.* 2004; **11**(2): 91–8.

Griffin E. *A First Look at Communication Theory.* 3rd ed. New York, NY: McGraw-Hill; 1997.

Hamilton SJ, Martin DJ. A framework for effective communication skills. *Extended version of Nursing Times.* 2007; **103**(48): 30–1.

Hargie O, Dickson D. *Skilled Interpersonal Communication: research, theory and practice.* 4th ed. London: Routledge; 2004.

Hargie O, editor. *The Handbook of Communication Skills.* 3rd ed. London: Routledge; 2006.

Kalisch BJ. What is empathy? *Am J Nurs.* 1973; **73**(9): 1548–52.

Kristin A, Elisabeth S. Emotional Intelligence: a review of the literature with specific focus on empirical and epistemological perspectives. *J Clin Nurs.* 2007; **16**(8); 1405–16.

McCabe C, Timmins F. *Communication Skills for Nursing Practice.* Basingstoke: Palgrave Macmillan; 2006.

McKay M, Davis D, Fanning P. *Messages: the communication skills book.* Oakland, CA: New Harbinger Publications Inc.; 2009.

Mercer SW, Reynolds W. Empathy and quality of care. *Br J Gen Pract.* 2002; **52**(Suppl. 1): S9–12.

Platt FW, Keller VF. Empathic communication: a teachable and learnable skill. *J Gen Intern Med.* 1994; **9**(4): 222–8.

Rodgers CR. *A Way of Being.* Boston: Houghton Mifflin; 1994.

Rogers C. *On Becoming a Person: a therapist's view of psychotherapy.* London: Constable; 1961.

Rose C. Taking authority in the group. *CPJ.* 2004; **16**(6): 43–5.

Rothwell JD. *In the Company of Others: an introduction to communication.* New York, NY: Oxford University Press; 2010.

Shattell MM, Starr SS, Thomas SP. Take my hand, help me out: mental health service recipients' experience of the therapeutic relationship. *Int J Ment Health Nurs.* 2007; **16**(4): 274–84.

Trevithick P, Richards S, Ruch G, *et al. Teaching and Learning Communication Skills in Social Work Education.* SCIE Knowledge Review 6. Bristol: Policy Press; 2004.

CHAPTER 6

Emotional intelligence and leadership

Derek Barron and John Hurley

As a student or recently qualified practitioner you may well be asking yourself why you should even be thinking about being a leader at this stage of your career. However, leadership in this sense is not about being 'in charge' or taking on all the responsibility for a department or ward. From the outset of your career you will be expected to possess and, more importantly, show leadership capabilities across academic, clinical and even social settings. While this may include leading other people for short periods of time or on a particular task, leadership applies as much to leading yourself as it does to leading other people. Understanding and applying EI to this concept will help you communicate to others that you have these leadership abilities and feel confident in demonstrating them.

This chapter applies EI to key aspects of leading self and others within contemporary health and social settings, which are often characterised by change and uncertainty. This view on leadership takes a particular focus upon what are called transformational, democratic and clinical leadership styles. We will also discuss the pivotal characteristics of something called collaborative individualism, a term that describes the way you achieve key parts of your role.

BACKGROUND

Within health and social care, leadership has historically been about being in charge of other staff, arranging and managing tasks to be completed and exercising some degree of power and hence control over others. Arguably, some leaders within those roles have not always been the most talented of leaders, often resorting to autocratic and militarised leadership approaches. Such views toward leadership mean that there are very few leaders, each with a small disparate army of followers. Defenders of such approaches will argue that throughout history the only constant within health and social care settings has been change, and that these highly directive leadership approaches undertaken by an elite few and supported by intensive management systems are the only way to get the job done. History perhaps suggests that while hitting the target, they frequently miss the point.

However, there are in fact ways of leading people and still getting the job done: this is true, even in big organisations. The National Health Service (NHS) across the United Kingdom is the largest organisation to be found in Europe and it has gone through significant periods of change, the most conspicuous one coming with devolution in 1999. This saw the end of (if it ever existed) a single vision of what the NHS should be and the underlying principles upon which services are delivered. Devolution brought a closer alignment between the individuality of party politics (notably those in power in each of the four home countries) and how services were run in each of the home countries. Within Scotland in particular it saw a greater politically driven focus on leadership within the NHS, as its chief executives and other top positions are appointed through a process that requires political approval. It also heralded, within a Scottish context, the return of healthcare based on values and clinical engagement; a system more focussed on clinical leadership than other areas of the UK. Within England in particular, professional managerialism emerged as the preferred way of getting health and social care to people.

Two points should hopefully be emerging as you read this; one is that there is a significant difference between being a leader and being a manager, a difference we will explore a little later. The second point is that the political systems of the country in which you work directly shape the services you work in, which in turn shapes the type of leadership expected of you in your professional roles. The NHS example within the UK highlights this. The NHS can be seen as delivering a market-driven economy loosely based on the principle of 'healthcare free at the point of delivery' (Greer 2004, Greer and Rowland 2008). However, Klein (2008) suggests: *'The NHS is a remarkable monument to institutional stability and political consensus. The old building has been massively remodelled, but the basic architecture remains intact'*. This professional managerialism creates a different focus from the professional clinical leadership more evident in the Scottish (and to a lesser extent the Welsh) system, which emphasise clinical autonomy, creativity and to an extent diversity built on clinical evidence and/or professional judgement.

Professional managerialism negatively impacts on the underlying principle of person-centredness and human rights, the foundation of the Scottish system and indeed Scottish mental health legislation (Mental Health (Care and Treatment) (Scotland) Act 2003, Millan principles SEHD 2004). Critically, systems such as those in Scotland also place on its managers and clinical leaders an irrevocable responsibility to work together to bring stated values into delivered values – a task not always achieved or even consistently achievable. It could be argued that less managed (as distinct from over-managed or unstructured) systems support this delivery of value-driven health and social care. Additionally, it is suggested that it also requires EI competent leaders focussed on people rather than simply on targets.

CONTEXT OF CHANGE

Regardless of your national context, health services have gone through, and continue to go through, significant and rapid cycles of change that require a high level of resilience from everyone. This change is not unrelated to the significant public finance investment it takes to run these systems as a proportion of the nation's entire budget. This leads to a semi-constant state of political flux related to the cycles of elections and political expedients of the government of the day. This issue of change provides a very important and common context in which health and social care leadership is situated. This resilience to the effects of organisational change is perhaps more important for the clinician as leader, who often does not manage services but is frequently required to influence without authority, while still being able to share and lead the vision of continuous improvement and deliver high-quality, person-centred care. Indeed, there can be few clinical leaders who have not gone through and had to cope with significant organisational restructurings (Dooley 2002).

The role of the emotionally intelligent leader can significantly mitigate the impact of these restructurings and workforce changes (Cummings *et al.* 2005). Cummings *et al.* (2005) found that leaders with what is called a 'resonant leadership' style reduced the negative emotional impact that change had on staff. Resonant leaders were empathetic and supportive to the needs of their teams while also effectively taking notice and control of their own emotions. They were able to manage and develop relationships with others through a strong sense of self-awareness and self-management. Cummings *et al.* (2005) describe some characteristics of the dissonant leader (as distinct from resonant) as *'pace setting and commanding'*; the dissonant leader destabilises the emotional underpinnings that support teams and deliver success. They frequently respond to change in a manner that 'burns out' their teams and ultimately the staffs within the teams do not own the innovation or changes, but rather feel imposed upon. As noted previously in this chapter, they hit the target, but miss the point. Health and social care services are about people – those we serve and those that do the serving; we ignore both at our peril. The dissonant leader's need to achieve the target overrides any understanding of the humanity of their teams or indeed the people they serve.

What must be understood here is that resonant leaders also deliver change and innovation and are often at the very forefront of development; it is the 'how' of delivery that is different. The resonant leader supports their staff to work through the change, to develop solutions, to own what is happening. Staff that are given ownership of change and have the ability to influence change frequently deliver more than was asked of them – often termed the discretionary effort. The sense of ownership impacts on the emotional well-being of teams and the individuals within the teams. Segal (2002) suggests that emotionally intelligent healthcare leaders not only contribute to the wellbeing of those that they come into contact with as part of their work, but also contribute to the overall wellbeing of the institution itself.

The resonant leader is not afraid to surround himself with people that know more than he does – it is not his role to know everything. Conversely, the dissonant leader has an unshakeable need to be the one that knows the answers, to be able to command and control both the direct and the pace of change. Within themselves they are frequently challenged by people who know more than they do.

LEADING SELF AND OTHERS

Good leadership with the health and social care setting has key characteristics in common with leadership in any sphere of work, for example:

- commitment to service excellence
- integrity
- approachability
- visionary ability
- visibility
- intelligence
- sound judgement
- decisiveness
- knowledge
- fluency
- personality
- adaptability
- alertness
- integrity
- non-conformity.

Good leadership does, however, have features that differentiate it from many other walks of life. Leadership within health and social care needs to inspire and motivate others within workplace environments characterised by expressed emotion, co-existing with the need to think rationally and creatively. Unlike most other walks of life, healthcare clinical leaders are dealing with life and death as well as risk and vulnerability as a day-to-day factor, consequently impacting on those using services, as well as those that deliver the services.

To a different extent leaders within social care also deal with life and vulnerability as central components of their day-to-day life. Contact with health and social services is, in the main, related to ill health or areas of health/care deficit – this impacts therefore on the underpinning emotion of the episode of engagement and the impact this can have on the staff dealing with that emotion. Although a recovery approach has emerged as the central philosophy of both health and social care service, this perspective acknowledges the underlying tenet that services are focussed on people during an illness or deficit stage of their life. The leader therefore has to deal with the emotion generated from those using the service as well as the emotion of staff providing the episode of care. Indeed, emotion and emotional engagement is threaded throughout the relationships that exist across health and social care, with the use of the personal/professional self being a key fundamental capability to achieving improved clinical and social outcomes (Lynch and Trenoweth 2008).

Perhaps by now you are asking the question – am I or would I be a dissonant leader? Am I the type of leader who through a drive to accomplish goals and tasks would not actually lead at all, but be in fact pushing? These questions direct us toward seeing leadership as being pertinent to all of us engaged in health and social care delivery, rather than applying only to an elite few. Leadership commences with leading ourselves and being a collaborative individual, a term we will expand upon shortly. By being able to lead ourselves we are in a much better place to respond to the key question asked of effective leaders: 'Why should I be led by you?' (Jumaa 2008).

Box 6.1   Reflection activity

Who would be your favourite or most respected leadership figure? Try and relate this to someone you have worked with or encountered in real life.

Write down at least six key characteristics of that leader. Include his/her values and attitudes as well as what he/she actually did.

Compare your list of key characteristics with the EI capabilities outlined in Chapter 1. Is there compatibility between the two?

Box 6.2   Reflection activity

Now write down six key characteristics of poor leaders you have encountered.

In comparing the characteristics of the good and bad leaders, what would you say are the underlying differences?

Finally (and perhaps the most important) reflective activity to undertake and respond to honestly in some depth is: 'in both your personal and professional roles how will you ensure you inspire people to believe in you as a leader?' Of great importance here is the recognition that 'leadership' is not a destination, it's not something you get promoted into, it exists at all levels in an organisation – it has been said before that an organisation with one leader is short on leadership.

YOU ARE THE NEW GENERATION OF LEADERS

As an undergraduate or recently qualified professional you will directly contribute to the way the job gets done within your own clinical or educational setting. You have real choice on how you as both leader and follower interact with those around you. This choice can be to continue the historically dubious ways of leading and following, or as we hope, to be part of building an expanding mass of professionals who truly lead, i.e. those who lead without the need to dictate or bully.

A building block in achieving this shift is to be a person centred and emotionally intelligent leader, rather than one who in future years relies solely on organisational rank. Alimo-Metcalfe and Alban-Metcalfe (2008) present significant evidence from their research that underlines the 'person centredness' of the good leader. They describe the central component of what they call the transformational leader as showing genuine concern for others. The transformational leader exerts an influence on those around them, often through strong role modelling of behaviours. She inspires others to new possibilities, and rather than focussing on what is wrong, she is more tuned to 'how to make things better'. The transformational leader draws out the strengths she has and communicates a vision of what might be; she takes an active part in building and maintaining the reality of that vision. The transformational leader looks to the future, but lives in the present.

Figure 6.1 helps us to picture that interrelatedness of self and others – leaders and followers.

The leader needs to own, understand and be aware of these internal emotions alongside the interpersonal emotions, i.e. those of others the leader is in touch with. It is the awareness of this interlinking that enables the leader to function effectively. It is also this awareness that enables the leader to effectively support his followers, without losing the 'detachment' (yet remaining engaged!) required to respond empathetically rather than sympathetically. Of note, however, is that the dimensions of 'intra' and 'inter' personal do not exist in isolation; the critical factor is the self-awareness, from which the others flow.

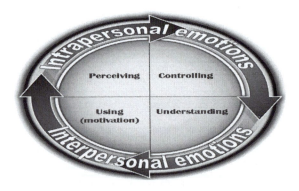

FIGURE 6.1 The interlinked aspects of intrapersonal emotions in leadership

Intrapersonal

The **perceiving** quadrant in Figure 1 relates to the leader's ability to self-reflect, to consider and to understand the impact he or she has on others. It is here the leader needs to understand his own emotions, especially in terms of why he is having that emotion at that particular time. She is aware of her own strengths and weaknesses and is able to take that awareness and use it to reflect on situations from the perspective of self-learning. Additionally, he is open to feedback from others. While some might find this a disconcerting task, once you accept that you, like those around you, are not perfect, and that you trust the person providing feedback, then it is a fantastic way to learn how to be a better leader; this does, however, require self-honesty as well as **self-control**. It requires an openness to one's own emotions and self-honesty in their management. The transformational and emotionally intelligent leader will also stay composed in the face of adversity – a situation all practitioners will face throughout their careers. It would be foolish to underestimate how difficult this can be at times; however the rewards, in terms of the leadership journey, are worth the effort. Unhelpful emotions are, unsurprisingly, the most challenging to address – human emotions such as disappointment, anger or anxiety also affect leaders, but it is what they do with these emotions that set them aside from others. Goleman, Boyatis and McKee (2002, p. 57) describe *'good hygiene'* as that ability, or indeed need, of the emotionally intelligent leader to deal with his or her own emotions through reflection. The leader has few opportunities to make a mistake with her own emotions before losing a level of credibility with followers.

Interpersonal

The interpersonal quadrants in Figure 1 relates to how we engage with others. At the very centre of **understanding** is the attribute of empathy. Empathy describes the ability to sense or feel what another person may be experiencing as if you were that person – the key is without losing the 'as if' quality. The following is an old tale to demonstrate this, which has been recited many times:

> Someone falls into a hole 10 feet deep. He has hurt his leg, it's cold and it's getting dark. To sympathise with him would be for you to jump into the hole with him, wrap a blanket round him and share words of comfort – before long you would be just as miserable, just as cold and unable to get out of the hole. To empathise with them you would be to call down to them, agree with them that it must be pretty rough stuck down there in the hole, that you understand how cold it must be and that they are in pain, you may throw a blanket down to them – then you can go and get the fire brigade to get a ladder and help them out.

This is an overly simplistic story to help demonstrate a complex concept. The emotionally intelligent or transformational leader with this attribute would be recognised by followers as approachable, while perceptive to the emotions of the follower – both positive and negative. She is able to remain attentive to the emotional cues of her teams, active listening is a skill at which she is adept. This demonstrates an understanding of the perspective of others and shows a sense of sensitivity to it.

In addition to being empathetic, EI leaders are able to develop those around them; they are able to recognise the strengths of others and to support the development of individuals and teams. They are able to see and 'read' relationships about them – this is important in terms of collaboration and on occasions conflict management. They support mutual understanding of issues through their tact and diplomacy; a key feature is their ongoing desire to achieve a win-win outcome from a situation (including conflicts). This approach is possible through a balance between the 'task' and an appropriate focus on relationships, through which they are able to build a rapport with others. They are able to spot opportunities for collaboration and develop these toward shared outcomes.

Motivating – in the exercise undertaken earlier in this chapter it is likely that you will have used the word 'motivating' in relation to one of the 'five key characteristics of good leaders you have encountered'. The EI leader inspires and motivates others to go beyond just doing the job. In engaging with those around them the leader doesn't simply empower them to reach beyond the norm to achieve extraordinary things; they inspire them to take that 'empowerment' for themselves – it becomes the norm, it is not something 'given', which of course can then be taken away. This inspirational motivation is not the charismatic, heroic leaders we can see quoted as 'saving companies' (Alimo-Metcalfe and Alban-Metcalfe 2005, Mintzberg 1999) – this 'charismatic/heroic' type of leadership is more frequently associated with self-promotion, which divides rather than builds bonds with others.

Goleman *et al.* (2002) regarded the above as traits and skills, whereas Mayer *et al.* (2004) talked about abilities that then cross over into personality. One could argue that these are semantics and in the real world of applying these there is little actual difference. What is more important is the question whether, unlike intelligence quotient (IQ), EI can be learnt – if EI skills and abilities can't be learnt or adapted, it raises many questions around the value of trying to teach leadership at any level in any organisation; indeed it could be asked why you would be reading this book. From the authors' personal experiences of working with nurses over several years, we are in no doubt that EI can be learnt. Some will always more skilled in its application than others, in much the way as any other skill where some will undoubtedly reach a higher level of proficiency than others.

Box 6.3   Reflection activity

Reflect on an experience of change you have witnessed – perhaps ward restructure or a community team redesign.
- Did the process simply focus on what was wrong?
- Did the process focus on the abilities of the team to deliver change?

Now consider this from a personal perspective. When you have been involved in planning care with someone, perhaps via a care plan – did you focus on the illness or deficit that caused the person to come into contact with the service, or did you focus on the strengths the individual had to assist them overcoming the deficit?

High achievement takes place in an environment of high expectation – if there is constant focus on the weakness/deficits of a team or individual the likelihood is those teams/individuals will simply live up to the expectations placed upon them, i.e. what they aren't able to do will become their own limiting self-belief.

EI health or social care leaders therefore work in an intensely emotional environment. They are role models within their services and teams. They demonstrate respect and co-operation for teams and individuals; they are consistent in their approach and approachability – they are also able to admit their mistakes, while being willing learners. Within the health and social care environment they are able to handle multiple tasks and interruptions to a range of changing priorities without losing the person at the centre of the care experience.

LEADERSHIP QUALITIES AND EMOTIONAL INTELLIGENCE

There are a number of qualities that staff associate with effective leadership and the use of EI. Ruderman *et al.* (2004) were able to identify 10 areas associated with EI and effective leadership; these are:

- **participative management**: getting buy-in from colleagues at the beginning of an initiative by involving them in the process and building consensus, engaging them through listening and communicating, influencing them in the decision-making
- **putting people at ease**: gets at the heart of making others relaxed and comfortable in your presence; provides meaningful engagement with others
- **self-awareness:** describes those managers who have an accurate understanding of their strengths and weaknesses; communicating and working within these; demonstrating a willingness to improve their own skills and capabilities
- **balance between personal life and work**: measures the degree to which work and personal life activities are prioritised so that neither is neglected; this is another way of demonstrating that the person is a capable manager
- **straightforwardness and composure:** refers to the skill of remaining calm in a crisis and recovering from mistakes; associated with stress tolerance, social responsibility and optimism (the ability to maintain a positive attitude even in the face of adversity)
- **building and mending relationships:** is the ability to develop and maintain working relationships with various internal and external parties and to negotiate work-related problems without alienating people

- **doing whatever it takes**: the leadership abilities of being perseverant and staying focused in the face of obstacles, of being action oriented and taking charge, and of taking a stand on one's own if required; whilst at the same time acknowledging and taking on board the views of others
- **decisiveness**: the ability to be self-directed and self-controlled in one's thinking
- **confronting problem employees**: the degree to which a manager acts decisively and fairly when dealing with problem employees, and the EI measure of assertiveness
- **change management**: the ability and effectiveness at implementing strategies to facilitate organisational change initiatives and overcome resistance to change.

The above factors make for interesting reading. Again, the importance of being self-aware is highlighted, as is need to be sensitive to the needs of others, even when getting the job done. There is also the sense of being in control, although this may not always be the case, and the need to portray and communicate this in our undertakings. It is suggested here that buy-in is not just into a project or initiative, but also the leader.

LEADING WITHIN TEAMS

With staff changes and organisational restructuring as part of our working practice, the implementation of integrated practice needs to become an inherent part of our work; one which requires active management and leadership. The professional background of workers can act as both a strength and a barrier to effective working across groups. As each profession has developed its own language and body of knowledge, it not only serves to provide a professional identity but can alienate those outside the profession who do not share their language or way of thinking. Professionals also work in different ways, following differing agendas and practices. Practitioners do not work in isolation but as part of multi-professional teams. For any practitioner, whether a medic, social worker, occupational therapist or nurse, there are three factors that will influence the practitioner's practice and use of EI; these include:

1   personal life history and what has motivated the practitioner to work in this chosen profession
2   professional background, training and experience
3   the agency in which he or she works and what the beliefs, values, aims and objectives of the agency are (Chandler 2006, p. 142).

EI allows the practitioner to lead and navigate these groups; taking account of how the different professionals view their own roles and bring them together through a common purpose and shared value base. Being mindful and taking account of these different ways of working is only the first step. Seeking genuine collaboration and consultation within groups is another.

Behaviours of an effective leader

- Think critically – choose actions clearly
- Solve problems
- Respect individuals
- Listen and communicate carefully and skillfully
- Set goals and a vision for the future
- Develop oneself and coach others

LEADING, FOLLOWING AND BEING COLLABORATIVE

To end this chapter we want to briefly look at the issue of followership. It may be self-evident that for someone to be a leader, there must be followers. This may on the surface seem self-explanatory; all I have to do to be a follower is to … follow the leader. However, this would merely create the type of leader–follower relationships we have described as being less effective and potentially dictatorial.

Limerick *et al.* (2002) offer an alternative to this old-fashioned way of following; they consider something called a collaborative individual. Rather than behaving like herded sheep, such followers are:

- autonomous
- interdependent
- proactive
- collaborative
- accountable
- communicative
- creative
- assertive.

Their values will match those of the organisations for which they work, and they will be able to not merely cope with change, but use change creatively. The authors' experiences as leaders within organisations are that the collaborative individual will come with not only the problematic issue, but the potential solution/s to that issue. He or she will work well with others and yet be equally adept at working alone.

Box 6.4 Reflection activity

Make a list of what intrapersonal capabilities, values and attitudes you would need to have to be a collaborative individual. For example, to be willing to relinquish control or to enact assertiveness would be two such capabilities.

You will clearly note that the abilities of the collaborative individual are well suited to not only being able to work in more traditional health and social care settings, but they are also highly valuable in providing community-based interventions. In these community settings you will be required to network with other organisations to meet all the needs of those that use your services. All these care providers will have both shared and simultaneously different values and priorities and even possibly professional language to your own. You will need to be able to lead your section of that care while working in effective collaboration with others. Hence, being able to communicate mutual respect, trust and authenticity are key capabilities to ensure effective collaborative working that in turn meets the needs of service consumers. These same abilities are also well suited to deal with the issue of unceasing change within services as discussed earlier in the chapter.

Finally, rather than providing a traditional summary of the chapter, this section will end with comments from current practitioners about EI and leadership.

- 'I believe EI is essential for any practitoner, not just managers and leaders. It provides valuable insight, enabling nurses to provide care in sometimes difficult and constantly changing situations.'
- 'It is vital then for leaders to develop and enhance their EI to successfully and effectively lead teams, particularly in this time of nursing shortages.'
- 'People/followers need to feel truly valued/respected, as individuals and leaders displaying EI are probably more successful.'
- 'I think that often leaders within the NHS are not portrayed as being empathetic on occasions and are just focussed on getting the job done. Incorporating EI will help leaders in becoming more influential and successful.'
- 'Awareness and utilisation of EI can be applied to any professional and personal interaction. We may work with others we personally may not like but require to have a professional relationship [with] to attain a goal, and an understanding of EI could assist this interaction.'
- 'Leaders should be aware of how they communicate, especially non-verbally: it can effect others' perceptions of them. For example, something as simple as a failure to smile or say hello can maybe cause a negative effect on others around you even when not done deliberately; leaving them thinking maybe incorrectly that you're unapproachable, unfriendly.'
- 'Being able to know, clarify and regulate your emotions and utilise them in an adaptive way to influence decisions, behaviour and relationships is important for us as individuals, practitioners and leaders. We spend a lot of time as nurses (and leaders) guiding others, supporting them to find the best way forward in difficult situations, etc. – and for this to happen, self-awareness on their behalf is needed.'
- 'Collective reform must first be individual reform. With this in mind I think it is vital to be able to reflect on our abilities and capabilities. These personal or "self" competencies would form part of the individual reform I mentioned.'
- 'We should lead by example. Hopefully all us enlightened souls can inspire and motivate others, and this could in some way guide their performance.'

REFERENCES

Alimo-Metcalfe B, Alban-Metcalfe J. Leadership: time for a new direction? *Leadership.* 2005; **1**(1): 51–71.

Alimo-Metcalfe B, Alban-Metcalfe J. *Engaging Leadership: creating organisations that maximise the potential of their people.* London: Chartered Institute of Personnel and Development; 2008.

Chandler T. Working in multidisciplinary teams. In: Pugh G, Duffy B, editors. *Contemporary Issues in the Early Years.* London: Sage Publications; 2006.

Cummings G, Hayduk L, Estabrooks C. Mitigating the impact of hospital restructuring on nurses: the responsibility of emotionally intelligent leadership. *Nursing Research.* 2005; **54**(1): 2–12.

Dooley K. Organisational complexity. In: Warner M, editor. *International Encyclopedia of Business and Management.* London: Thompson Learning; 2002. pp. 5013–22.

Goleman D, Boyatzis R, McKee A. The emotional reality of teams. *Journal of Organizational Excellence.* 2002; **21**(2): 55–65.

Greer S. *Four Way Bet: how devolution has led to four different models for the NHS.* London: The Constitution Unit; 2004.

Greer S, Rowland D. *Devolving Policy, Diverging Values? The values of the United Kingdom's National Health Services.* England: The Nuffield Trust; 2008.

Jumaa M, Marrow C. Nursing leadership development: why should any nurse be lead by you? *J Nurs Manag.* 2008; **16**(8): 893–7.

Klein R. What does the future hold for the NHS at 60? *BMJ.* 2008; **337**: 1–2.

Limerick D, Cunnington B, Crowther F. *Managing the New Organisation: collaboration and sustainability in the post-corporate world.* 2nd ed. Crows Nest, NSW: Allen & Unwin; 2002.

Lynch J, Trenoweth S, editors. *Contemporary Issues in Mental Health Nursing.* Chicester: John Wiley and Sons; 2008.

Mayer J, Salovey P, Caruso D. Emotional intelligence: theories, findings and implications. *Psychological Inquiry.* 2004; **15**(3): 197–215.

Mintzberg H. Managing quietly. *Leader to Leader.* 1999; **12**(Spring): 24–30.

Ruderman MN, Hannum K, Brittain J, *et al.* Making the Connections: leadership skills and EI. In: Wilcox M, editor. *The CCL Guide to Leadership in Action: how managers and organizations can improve the practice of leadership.* New York, NY: Jossey-Bass; 2004.

Scottish Executive Health Department. *The Mental Health (Care and Treatment) (Scotland) Act 2003: a short introduction.* Edinburgh: Scottish Executive Health Department; 2004.

Segal J. Good leaders use 'emotional intelligence'. Emotionally intelligent leadership is a skill that can be learned and taught throughout life. *Health Progress.* 2002; **83**(3): 44–46, 66.

CHAPTER 7

Using emotional intelligence to navigate a critical incident

Paul Linsley and Nigel Horner

Practitioners of all backgrounds have come to appreciate the usefulness of EI in understanding their own as well as other people's behaviour and responses to challenging situations. This chapter, and the one that follows, looks at how EI may be used to manage and make sense of emotionally charged incidents and occurrences in clinical practice. Whilst the two chapters focus on emotional touchpoints – in other words, points of emotional vulnerability – the underlying principles and approaches discussed hold good regardless the situation the practitioner might find him- or herself in. Within these two chapters, the need for emotional sensitivity and critical reflection are highlighted, as is the willingness to engage in emotional dialogue with self and colleagues. This understanding is a necessary component of all healthcare interventions and recognises the individual nature and uniqueness of people and their circumstances.

CRITICAL INCIDENTS

As part of their daily work, practitioners are frequently faced with problems and incidents that have to be contained, managed and resolved. They will meet people who are going through the most traumatic of times, which may have a variety of happy and sad outcomes. Often, practitioners will deal with these incidents without giving much thought as to how they managed the situation and with little regard to their emotional and psychological well-being; 'It's just part of the job'. However, there are times when these incidents become critical and challenge the person's ability to cope and deal with matters. Something that seemed trivial one day can be 'blown out of proportion' the next and poorly handled. These incidents can place considerable stress on those that have to deal with them and those that have to subsequently mange and support them.

'Incidents happen, but critical incidents are produced by the way we look at a situation: a critical incident is an interpretation of the significance of an event. To take something as a critical incident is a value judgement we make, and the basis of the judgement is the significance we attach to the meaning of the incident.' (Tripp 1993, p. 8, reproduced with permission of Taylor and Francis Group LLC-Books)

Incidents become critical incidents when those involved attach a particular significance to them (Chell 1998) and as such, are subject, time and context specific. Critical incidents' environments are often characterised by high time pressure, incomplete information and changing circumstances (Alison and Crego 2008, Flin and Arbuthnot 2002) (*see* Figure 7.1), all factors which contribute to how we perceive and subsequently manage events. Navigating such environments requires the person to quickly process information and events, take appropriate action, and be mindful of their own, and others', well-being.

> ### Stress within the workplace
>
> Emotional unease and stress within the workplace frequently originates from:
> - time pressure, work overload, role uncertainty and role conflict (Antonioni and Park 2001)
> - selection and placement of employees without considering individual stress (Robbins *et al.* 1998)
> - unattainable goal setting, minimal goal feedback, job design not matching employee capacity and exclusive decision-making (Robbins *et al.* 1998).

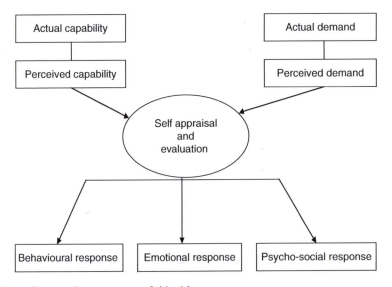

FIGURE 7.1 Responding to a stressful incident

The initial response to a critical incident tends to be a physiological one, with high levels of arousal and emotional upset. The person may be responding to external demands, such as keeping control of the situation, and it may be some time before the person starts to make sense of what has happened to him or her. This initial set of reactions can include psychological shock, numbness, confusion, disorientation and a feeling of bewilderment. Often people will ask: 'Could I have done things differently?' or 'Was I to blame for the incident?' Reactions will vary from individual to individual; however, here are some of the common reactions and responses to incidents that challenge our emotional well-being (*see also* Boyce *et al.* 2001, Parkinson 1997, O'Driscoll and Cooper 1996):

- **shock:** a disbelief that the event has happened or is happening
- **fear:** that the situation might escalate or happen again; our sense of safety and security is challenged
- **anger:** a psychological response to a situation, which may be inwardly directed towards the self or outwardly towards others; it is dependant on who the person sees as being responsible for what happened or is happening
- **sadness:** can exist about anything but may be centred on loss, grief and concerns for safety
- **a sense of injustice:** 'This should never have happened'
- **shame and guilt:** the individual may feel that he is somehow to blame for what happened or what is taking place, that he did not behave as he should have or did not do as much as he could have
- **frustration:** at not being able to change or undo things: a perceived delay in help, services and support.

In turn, how an individual responds to a critical incident will depend on a number of factors; some of which are listed below (*see also* Thompson 2004, Paton 2003, Vettor and Kosinski 2000):

- **control over the incident:** a sense of being out of control can heighten anxiety and lead to confusion; the more in control the person feels the better able he or she is to manage
- **predictability:** was the event expected or totally 'out of the blue'?
- **control over duration:** 'Was there something we could have done better?' 'Could we have been more prepared?'
- the way the person **interprets** what has happened
- feelings of **competency** or **incompetency**
- **emotional self-control:** the extent of control the person has over his or her emotions
- **past life events:** past losses, inabilities, history of failure, etc. may make the person more vulnerable to what is happening in the here and now.

The important thing is to remember that these are normal responses to abnormal circumstances or events. Discussing the event without laying blame and allowing time to come to terms with what has happened can help in the recovery process. Staff may require support and encouragement to do this. Validation that things can and do go wrong, despite clinical competence and appropriate interventions, may also need to be stressed. Whatever support is offered should provide a means by which the person can work through his or her feelings and start to make sense of what happened. A sense of self-efficiency can be generated through a supportive professional development programme where staff members have the skills, knowledge and opportunities to work effectively and learn as part of the job.

MANAGING AND MAKING SENSE OF A CRITICAL INCIDENT USING EMOTIONAL INTELLIGENCE

Sama (1984) suggested that a critical incident can be thought of as having three stages or events; these are the:
1 **response phase** (threat, evaluation and containment)
2 **resolution phase** (contingency management)
3 **recovery phase** (restoration of normality).

The first stage requires the person to perceive and recognise warning signs of the evolving crisis. The second stage involves processing information to identify problems and causes and seeking out alternative ways of managing the situation, then putting these solutions into action and evaluating their success or otherwise. The third stage encourages a return to normality and a learning of lessons.

In addition to the above, Flin (1996 p. 37) identified three skills common to individuals who deal with critical incidents effectively; these are: being able to cope with stress, decision-making and team management. These skills, Manner (2008) argued, require qualities and values that run deeper than one's capacity and willingness to deal with such incidents effectively, but require EI in order to bring about a successful conclusion. Furthermore, these qualities and values are informed and developed, depending on one's personality, life experiences and personal influences.

The role of EI in managing a critical incident should be viewed in two dimensions:
1 the practitioners' perception and understanding of their and others' emotions and their behaviour in response to these, and
2 the management and utilisation of these perceptions to achieve the goal of making sense and managing the situation as it presents.

This requires the management of a number of factors, including the person's level of competence and experience; the resources available to the staff member at the time of the incident (staffing levels and other tasks that need completing), and the requirements of the organisation for which the individual works. In order to do this the person needs to mindful of how they and others are functioning and responding to the situation as it unfolds. Sensitivity of this kind requires emotional monitoring of the environment and a preparedness to intervene and take action based on sound decision-making. The use of EI in these incidences encourages the promotion of positive attitudes, greater adaptability and flexibility in tackling the situation and an increased orientation towards positive values (Kristin and Elisabeth 2007). In this sense EI can be seen as a navigation tool by which the person orientates him- or herself to the situation and then plans actions based upon value systems and ways of working that reflect professional competence and thinking.

Whilst Goleman (1995) developed his model of EI (*see* Chapter 1, Introducing emotional intelligence) with direct reference to leadership qualities, it also provides a useful means for navigating and making sense of critical incidents. The first of Goleman's (1995) four-stage model is the need to be self-aware. If we refer back to Tripp's (1993) definition of a critical incident at the beginning of the chapter, we are reminded that a critical incident is 'an interpretation of the significance of an event'. We often feel at a loss as to what is happening and question our ability to cope. The first stage then to managing a critical incident is to regain control of our thoughts and emotions and channel them in a more constructive way. A person with a high degree of EI would be one who responded to situations with feeling states that 'made good sense', given what was going on in these situations. Appropriately generated feeling states would serve as a motivator to pursue reasonable behaviour or action.

In order to do this, the practitioner needs to learn to identify shifts in arousal levels and use these as a measure as to how they are coping and, if things are beginning to 'get out of hand', bring them under control again. By failing to monitor and manage their emotions, a person runs the risk of acting impulsively and making decisions based on disruptive and irrational patterns of thinking and feeling rather than clarity and control of thought. The use of relaxation techniques, and in particular controlled breathing, are advocated here as a means of regaining these.

Emotional resilience of the kind described above plays an important factor in the way we perceive events and our capabilities to manage the situations that we find ourselves in. The use of self-awareness and self-analysis has been suggested as being particularly relevant to healthcare practitioners due to the nature of their work – the need to respond to individual requirements and needs of clients, and to avoid rigid routines of caring acts that can lead to performing duties on 'autopilot' (Cox 1994). It also allows creative thinking and problem-solving and encourages flexibility of response to challenging and demanding situations.

Recognising one's emotions and managing their effects instils a sense of purpose, a regaining of control. Situational awareness of 'gut feelings' can further enhance this process and give confidence to act; this innate ability is important as it draws on past experience and ways of coping. Being aware of your emotions during an escalating event can help the person to avoid indecisiveness and help promote confidence in others as well as an understanding of what is happening.

A person's usual ways of coping are challenged during a critical incident (*see* Figure 7.1) and may prove ineffective in dealing with the situation. An accurate self-assessment, knowing one's strengths and limits, and acting within those limits, can help to safeguard personal and professional integrity.

Knowing when to access help and support is also important. Sometimes, just articulating your thoughts and feelings as to how to manage a situation can be helpful. The following three statements may prove insightful:
- here's what I think we face (assessment of the situation)
- here's what I think we should do (option appraisal)
- here's why (evidence base).

From these the practitioner can develop a plan of coping as well as a plan of action and allocate or seek resources and support as appropriate. The trick here is to bide yourself some time in which to make sense of what is happening and feeling, looking for possible reasons as to why you might be responding to the situation as you are.

The second phase of Goleman's model (1995), self-management refers to managing internal emotional states, impulses and personal resources. Important here is the keeping of disruptive emotions and thoughts in check and not allowing them to drive and shape the decisions that you make. Our internal dialogues play an important role in shaping and defining our emotional experiences and can prove disruptive, particularly when in a stressful situation. Such thoughts tend to be overly critical in nature and it is this that distorts constructive thinking. Thoughts that are irrational in nature need to be safeguarded against, and a proper and thorough appraisal of the situation needs to be undertaken. Focus should be on problem-solving techniques and tackling the situation as it presents.

In portraying conscientiousness, there is a need to take responsibility for personal performance and maintaining standards of honesty and integrity in keeping with professional standards and codes of conduct as well as being true to ourselves and what we believe in. Sometimes we feel uncomfortable with stepping outside of our 'safety zone' and are rigid in how we approach situations; flexibility in thought and action is recommended, as is embracing new and innovative ways of working. This does not mean a compromise of standards but a willingness to view things in a different way, recognising that whilst others may be experiencing similar feelings toward the situation, they may have a different view as to how it should be managed. Problem-solving is a useful approach here as it allows the person to not only manage staff but emotions. The key is to reframe the thoughts that underpin a particular situation in emotional terms and to see the issue afresh, e.g.:
- 'the real problem isn't what's done that bothers me; the problem is how I feel'
- 'the real problem isn't why it happened; the real problem is why I responded the way I did'.

The third phase of Goleman's model (1995) is social awareness. In terms of managing a critical incident, this is the monitoring and management of others and responding to their needs in relationship to what you are going through and experiencing. This requires a great deal of sensitivity and a desire to help support others. Social competence and professional etiquette are challenged, and the way we manage and handle relationships is scrutinised. Expect that staff will have various emotions and reactions to any given situation or event. Reading a group's emotional currents can help navigate a situation to a successful conclusion. Be alert to what is going on in the workplace and have some idea about how you will respond. Drawing on others' strengths and experiences can also bolster our own coping strategies as well as energise those around us into tackling the problem, through the installation of a sense of moving things forward. Important here is the need to put the client first. Anticipating, recognising and meeting a minimum level of client activity and service provision can provide a helpful basis on which to make decisions and centre discussion with team members.

However, staff experiences of work situations will and do vary between individual workers, even in similar situations. How client behaviour is interpreted, for example, the way in which it is defined, the meaning that is attached to it and the response it evokes are primarily dependent on staff perceptions. This might lead to a situation where one member of staff considers certain client behaviour as indicative of defensiveness, while another sees it as irrational behaviour. It is therefore important to be aware of the subjective and varied nature of these perceptions in assessing the behaviour of clients and their relatives. For example, the healthcare worker who considers the expression of anger or aggression inappropriate will approach an agitated patient differently from the other who considers agitated behaviour to be meaningful.

The fourth stage of Goleman's Emotional Intelligence Model (Goleman 1995) requires the practitioner not only to be sensitive to the needs of others but to lead and shape services. A critical incident may provide opportunities as well as challenges for change in ways of working, depending on the situation. It may, for instance, highlight a service need or new way of working. This adeptness to induce desirable responses and changes in services requires the following:

- **communication:** listening openly and sending convincing messages
- **conflict management:** negotiating and resolving disagreements
- **leadership:** inspiring and guiding individuals and groups
- **change catalyst:** initiating or managing change
- **building bonds:** nurturing instrumental relationships
- **collaboration and cooperation:** working with others towards shared goals
- **team capabilities:** creating group synergy in pursuing collective goals
- **providing feedback and encouragement:** acting as an ambassador for change
- **planning and problem solving:** assisting people facilitating solutions through the use of EI
- **information sharing:** that is relevant and useful to staff
- **modelling the values of the organisation:** for example, acting in a caring and thoughtful manner

- **initiative:** a readiness to act on opportunities as they present
- **optimism:** persistence in pursuing goals despite obstacles and setbacks.

The above are all things that can be employed to manage yourself and others in a critical incident. However, the degree to which these strategies can be utilised will be somewhat governed by the context in which the person works. Systems of support and ways of working need to be promoted so that staff members are able to explore their feelings and thoughts in a safe and confidential manner. Encouraging staff to share their concerns and problems and learn from mistakes is no mean feat, particularly in high-pressured environments where every second counts. Not allowing staff the opportunity, however, to pursue concerns can lead to mistakes being repeated. Encouraging the use of EI as part of a risk prevention strategy may help reduce the number of critical incidents within an area of work or enable people to look more constructively at these and learn from what has happened.

Box 7.1   Reflective activity

Emotional Intelligence consists of five key skills when managing a critical incident, each building on the last:
- the ability to quickly reduce stress
- the ability to recognise and manage your emotions
- the ability to connect with others using emotional sensitivity and resilience
- the ability to deal with challenges
- the ability to resolve conflicts positively and with confidence.

Take some time to reflect on what these competencies mean and assess yourself against them. From this you will be able to identity those areas that you need to concentrate on developing.

THE IMPORTANCE OF BECOMING A REFLECTIVE PRACTITIONER

Reflective practice allows the practitioner to consciously consider their experiences through integration of theory with practice, and in turn with praxis through experience.

'It is not sufficient simply to have an experience in order to learn. Without reflecting upon this experience it may quickly be forgotten, or its learning potential lost. It is from the feelings and thoughts emerging from this reflection that generalisations or concepts can be generated. And it is generalisations that allow new situations to be tackled effectively.' (Gibbs 1988, reproduced with permission of Oxford Brookes University)

Reflection involves defining a problem, asking questions, examining evidence, analysing assumptions and biases, confronting emotional unease, considering other interpretations, and tolerating ambiguity. It requires constructing new knowledge and new ways of thinking by perceiving a dilemma, exploring the differing perspectives, integrating existing knowledge and considering new alternatives. Reflection can be undertaken on an individual basis or through clinical supervision. Moon (1999) describes the process of reflection as a mental process which allows the person to make sense of complex ideas and thoughts.

Tripp (1993) suggests that by focusing on critical incidents in a structured and analytical way, we can develop our own 'grounded theory', i.e. explanations based on the collection and analysis of data. Used collaboratively and as part of action research (data gathering, wider reflection, action and evaluation), practitioners could develop increased understanding and control over professional judgements.

Self-assessment of this kind helps individuals reflect in a constructive way by 'returning to an experience, describing it and attending to thoughts and feelings' (Platzer *et al.* 1997, p. 193). Critical incident analysis is a structured form of reflection that seeks to measure practice and actions taken in a critical incident against professional codes of conduct and practice guidelines (Wilshaw and Bohannan 2003). The Critical Incident Technique involves:

- describing an incident from your recent professional experience that was either challenging or thought-provoking
- suggesting an explanation within the immediate context
- asking questions that delve deeper into the meaning behind the incident, e.g. different ways of thinking about it, exploring the dilemma, and considering personal theories and values, which influence that judgement
- considering the implications that this has for future practice (adapted from Tripp 1993).

The cognitive processes involved within self-assessment are complex; involving emotional evaluation and problem-solving (Moore 1998). In *Learning by Doing*, Gibbs (1988) outlines the stages for a 'Structured Debriefing', which is based on Kolb's (1984) Experiential Learning Cycle and encourages deeper reflection and self-analysis of the type described here:

Description

What is the stimulant for reflection, i.e. the incident? What are you going to reflect on? Describe the event in the sequence that it happened. What caused the event to happen as it did? What were the significant background factors to this experience?

Feelings

What were your reactions and feelings?

Evaluation

What was good and bad about the experience? Make value judgements.

Analysis

What sense can you make of the situation?
- What was I trying to achieve?
- Why did I intervene as I did?
- What were the consequences of my actions for myself and others?
- How did I feel about the experience when it was happening?
- How did others feel about it? How do I know how they felt?
- What factors/knowledge influenced my decisions and actions?

Bring in ideas from outside the experience to help you. Ask yourself, what was really going on?

Conclusions (general)

What can be concluded, in a general sense, from these experiences and the analyses you have undertaken?

Conclusions (specific)

What can be concluded about your own specific, unique, personal situation or ways of working?

Personal action plans

What are you going to do differently in this type of situation next time? What steps are you going to take on the basis of what you have learnt?

Adapting Gibbs for use in the immediacy of clinical practice

Casement (1985) suggests that healthcare professionals develop their own supervision within themselves, called the internal supervisor. Developing the ability to process helping interventions at the same time as engaging in them is a requirement of the effective healthcare practitioner. With a slight adaptation, the above model of self-analysis can be used in the immediacy of a situation to focus on how and why we are thinking and behaving as we are. An important part of internal supervision is 'trail identifying', this means putting yourself in the position of another in order to monitor your own part in what is happening. Changing the emphasis of the questions posed above allows navigation of this process in a structured and ordered way. Being self-aware and reflecting in this way allows a person to analyse his or her own feelings, beliefs and values through everyday situations. Furthermore, being honest with yourself about your self-doubts, abilities and personal limitations can help reduce 'personal pressures' of having to do some things well, each and every time (Dexter and Walsh 1995).

EMOTIONAL INTELLIGENCE AND SOCIAL WORK PRACTICE: A REFLECTIVE COMMENTARY

Here Nigel Horner provides a reflective commentary as to a challenge facing the social work profession and how EI may be play a part in meeting this.

This reflective piece looks at social work in terms of its capacity to engage with service users in an era of technical rationality. In the opinion of many commentators, social work appears to be a critical watershed of uncertainty, awaiting the final outcomes of the Munro Report entitled *Social Work, The Munro Review of Child Protection – Part One: a systems analysis* (Department of Education 2010) and the implementation of the 15 recommendations of the Social Work Taskforce (2009). To others, such a state is ever thus, arguing that social work is always a contingent activity, shaped by its particular political context, the conditions, concerns and peculiarities of its times (Harris 2008). In such an accepted environment of ambiguity, yet others search for the elements of an essential practice that transcends time and space. It is through this search that some argue that the essence of social work can be best understood by reference to the core characteristics required for effective engagement with those most vulnerable of individuals in the most complex and challenging circumstances.

By way of offering an all-too-rare appreciation of inherent complexities and expertise required for effective practice, the Department of Education (2010, p. 54) has stated:

> 'Social workers build relationships with children, young people and parents in extraordinarily difficult circumstances, and within a context that would appear from the outset to be counter to any chance of creating a positive dialogue … the children's social worker is frequently required to work with both parent and child in an extremely complex mix of hostility and psychological disorder.'

Faced with such a daunting prospect in any comparable professional sphere – building a bridge, defusing a bomb, developing a computer programme, performing a triple heart bypass – the reasonable question could be asked: how does the professional develop sufficient expertise to 'master' the situation?

The above are examples of expertise required to perform complex tasks utilising high-level skills, but all are performed in relation to either inanimate objects (the bridge, the bomb, the computer) or to normally sentient human beings under the abnormal conditions of an anaesthetic, which similarly makes the situation non-interactive.

By contrast, all social work situations are interactive, and all are therefore predicated upon the interpersonal capabilities of the practitioner. Whilst consistently acknowledged to be central to the helping process, the Munro Report observed that earlier reforms (of the child protection system) had 'tended to focus on technical solutions – increasing rules, more detailed procedures, more use of ICT – while giving less attention to the skills to engage with families, the expertise to bring about enduring improvements in parental behaviour, and the organisational support that enables social workers and others to manage the emotional dimensions of the work without it harming their judgement or their own well-being' (Department of Education 2010, p. 7).

What is being described here is the necessity for social work environments to promote and engender emotionally intelligent practice. So how is the term 'Emotional Intelligence' applied to social work practice? According to David Howe, EI is key to managing the stressful dynamics in fraught and highly charged situations, ranging from assessing children's situations in terms of safeguarding to facilitating the discharge of people from hospital following life-changing events and crises. 'Emotionally intelligent social workers help contain service users and their feelings in a relationship that feels safe – safe enough for them to explore. Workers who do not have these skills or agencies that come across as anxious, defensive or hostile alienate service users. Such agencies and their workers increase distress and anger' (Howe 2008, p. 182).

EI is about being tuned in to the complex and confused emotions of those bound up in a dramatic situation, including the service user, carers, other family members, as well as the practitioner and other professionals. As Morrison (2006, p. 59) notes: 'Once we are aware of our emotions we will be able to use these along with our knowledge and values to inform our practice. EI is not just about emotions, it encompasses a range of areas relating to the self and others [including] … assessment, help and care for others, advocacy [and] anxiety in times of crisis'.

The quality of decision-making in social work has long been under periodic attack. Every child death tragedy calls forth further degrees of incredulity about the various practitioners' apparent inability to apply cool, dispassionate logic to perceive the level of danger and thus to make the 'right' decisions regarding the child's safety and well-being. Whilst it has often been suggested that emotions cloud judgement, we would argue the opposite: that awareness and reflection upon one's own emotions are crucial to getting into the domain of practice wisdom, where the practitioner can use and integrate objective knowledge (concerning the child's weight, general health, growth patterns, educational performance, observable behaviours) alongside a subtle intuitive connection to what is being unsaid, what is not being revealed, what is the meta-dynamic of this family. As human beings, we have emotional responses to everything we work with: such is the consequence of being human. Such emotions can be seen as a 'destructive force overriding sound judgement' (Matthews 2002, p. 235) or a source of knowledge that needs to be embraced and understood.

Awareness of the emotional content of social work practice sits comfortably and consistently with current social work principles such as the promotion of service user involvement in the services they receive, but also in work with involuntary clients (Trotter 1999), where emotions are most highly charged in the context of potential threats to liberty and the sovereignty of private lives. A number of studies have shown that the greatest source of stress for social work practitioners arises not from interactions with service users – however complex they may be – but from frustrations with their organisational systems. Barlow and Hall (2007) refer this as 'moral distress', when a social worker wants to do something that he or she considers the correct thing to do but the organisation does not allow this to happen. It has been observed that EI has as much to do with knowing when and how to express emotion as it does with controlling it, and this certainly applies to the complex dynamics of inter-professional, multi-disciplinary practice that drives all service delivery arenas in the modern social work landscape.

Nevertheless, we would wish to assert and affirm a 50-year-old aphorism from one of the founders of casework, Father Biestek, who suggested that: 'One of the essentials in treating others is understanding and facing ourselves' (Biestek 1961, p. 28). Critically engaged practice is emotional: 'If you share the distress of people then you cannot walk away' (Dalrymple and Burke 1995, p. 1). As the Munro report possibly marks a turning of the tide away from technical rationality and mechanistic case management to a reaffirmation of the centrality of relationships at the heart of professional effectiveness, the concept of EI will prove to be central to the reclaiming of social work.

CONCLUSION

Critical incidents are those that challenge and extend the person's normal way of coping and dealing with matters. They are normal reactions to abnormal events. EI can be seen as a means of making sense of the situation and can help in the management of the event as it unfolds by promoting appropriate responses and ways of working. It should be recognised that emotional competencies are not mere innate talents, but learned capabilities that must be developed over time. The ability of the practitioner to perceive and reason, as well as the capacity to interact and respond to the emotional needs of others within challenging and demanding environments is an essential factor in promoting positive clinical outcomes.

REFERENCES

Alison L, Crego J, editors. *Policing Critical Incidents: leadership and critical incident management.* Devon: Willan Publishing; 2008.

Antonioni D, Park H. The effects of personality similarity on contextual work behaviours. *Person Psychol.* 2001; **54**: 331–360.

Barlow C, Hall B. 'What about feelings?': a study of emotion and tension in social work field education. *Social Work Education.* 2007; **26**(4): 399–413.

Biestek F. *The Casework Relationship.* London: Allen and Unwin; 1961.

Boyce P, Condon J, Stallard P, *et al.* Psychological debriefing. *BMJ.* 2001; **322**: 928.

Casement PJ. The internal supervisor. In: Casement PJ. *On Learning from the Patient.* London: Tavistock Publications; 1985.

Casement PJ. Internal supervision in process. In: Casement PJ. *Learning from Life: becoming a psychoanalyst.* London: Routledge; 2006.

Chell E. Critical incident technique. In: Symon G, Cassell C, editors. *Qualitative Methods and Analysis in Organizational Research.* London: Sage; 1998. pp. 51–72.

Clarke B. *Whose Life is It Anyway?* [play] 1981.

Cox S. Reflection and student learning. In: Gibbs G, editor. *Improving Student Learning.* Oxford: Oxford Centre for Staff Development; pp. 359–70.

Dalrymple J, Burke B. *Anti-Oppressive Practice.* Buckingham: Open University Press; 1995.

Dexter G, Walsh M. *Psychiatric Nursing Skills: a patient-centred approach.* London: Chapman and Hall; 1995.

Flin R. *Sitting in the Hot Seat: leaders and teams for critical incident management.* West Sussex: John Wiley & Sons Ltd.; 1996.

Flin R, Arbuthnot K. *Incident Command: tales from the hot seat.* Aldershot: Ashgate; 2002.

Gibbs G. *Learning by Doing: a guide to teaching and learning methods.* Oxford: FEU; 1988.

Goleman D. *Emotional Intelligence: why it can matter more than IQ.* 10th ed. New York, NY: Bantam Books; 1995.

Harris J. State social work: constructing the present from moments in the past. *Br J Soc Work.* 2008; **38**: 387–403.

Howe D. *The Emotionally Intelligent Social Worker.* Basingstoke: Palgrave Macmillan; 2008.

Kemppainen JK. The critical incident technique and nursing care quality system. *J Adv Nurs.* 2000; **32**(5): 1264–71.

Kolb D. *Experiential Learning: experience as the source of learning and development.* Upper Saddle River, NJ: Prentice Hall; 1984.

Kristin A, Elisabeth S. Emotional Intelligence: a review of the literature with specific focus on empirical and epistemological perspectives. *J Clin Nurs.* 2007; **16**(8); 1405–16.

Manner M. *Critical Incidents: effective responses and the factors behind them.* Nottingham: National College for School Leadership; 2008.

Matthews G. *Emotional Intelligence: science and myth.* Cambridge, MA: MIT Press; 2002.

Moon J. *Learning Journals: a handbook for academics, students and professional development.* London: Kogan Page; 1999.

Moore P. *Development of Professional Practice Research Training Fellowships: occasional papers.* Cardiff: Health Professions Wales; 1998.

Morrison T. Emotional intelligence, emotion and social work: context, characteristics, complications and contributions. *Br J Soc Work.* 2007; **37**(2): 245–63.

Munro E. *The Munro Review of Child Protection, Part One: a systems analysis.* London: Department of Education; 2010.

O'Driscoll MP, Cooper CL. A critical incident analysis of stress-coping behaviors at work. *Stress Medicine.* 1996; **12**: 123–8.

Parkinson F. *Critical Incident Debriefing: understanding and dealing with trauma.* London: Souvenir Press (E&A) Ltd.; 1997.

Paton D. Managing critical incident stress risk: a proactive approach. *Forum.* 2003; **8**: 36–40.

Platzer H, Blake D, Snelling J. A review of research into the use of groups and discussion to promote reflective practice in nursing. *Research in Post-Compulsory Education.* 1997; **2**(2): 193–204.

Robbins SP, Billet B, Cacioppe R, Waters-Marsh T. *Organisational Behaviour: Leading and Managing in Australia and New Zealand.* 2nd edition. Sydney: Prentice Hall; 1998.

Sama P. Training police commanders and supervisors in the management of critical incidents. *Washington Crime News Service, Training Aids Digest.* 1984; **9**(12): 1–6.

Social Work Task Force. *Building a Safe and Confident Future: the final report of the Social Work Task Force.* Available at: www.dcsf.gov.uk/swtf (accessed 17 July 2011).

Thompson R. Peer support: strategic response to intrastate incidents, remote deployment campaigns and community support. *Forum.* 2004; **8**: 5–28.

Tripp D. *Critical Incidents in Teaching: developing professional judgement.* London and New York: Routledge; 1993.

Tripp D. Teachers' lives, critical incidents and professional practice. *Qualitative Studies in Education.* 1994; **7**(1): 65–76.

Trotter C. *Working with Involuntary Clients.* London: Sage; 1999.

Vettor SM, Kosinski FA. Work-stress burnout in emergency medical technicians and the use of early recollections. *Journal of Employment Counseling.* 2000; **37**: 216–28.

Wilshaw G, Bohannon N. Reflective practice and team teaching in mental health care. *Nurs Stand.* 2003; **17**(50): 33–7.

CHAPTER 8

Emotional intelligence and the concept of emotional touchpoints in healthcare

Natalie Liddle

Editors' Note:

The following chapter builds on the ideas and concepts of Chapter 7 and is written by Natalie Liddle, a second-year nursing student at the University of Lincoln. Whilst Natalie writes from the perspective of her chosen profession, as with many of the ideas in this book, these are transferable and can be used by a range of healthcare practitioners as part of their clinical practice. The chapter will explore the relationship between EI, emotional labour and emotional touchpoints, or points of emotional vulnerability. Readers will be particularly drawn to explore how such concepts are currently being developed and used within healthcare.

INTRODUCTION

Emotional intelligence has been extensively explored, and many different paradigms exist within the social psychology literature (Cherniss 2002). Recently, such discussion and research has begun to take place within the context of health and social care and, in particular, within nursing (Cadman and Brewer 2001, Evans and Allen 2002, Freshman and Rubino 2002). EI has previously been considered to be an asset within certain professions where it is implicit to understand the views and emotions of others, which in turn enables professionals to become effective managers in practice (Vitello-Cicciu 2001). Furthermore, the use of EI in healthcare has been seen as crucial to the development of effective and meaningful relationships between patients and professionals (Freshwater and Stickley 2004).

This is supported by others who believe that the ability to recognise the emotional state of another is a prerequisite for those within the caring profession (Cadman and Brewer 2001). EI, therefore, seems a relevant and yet contemporary concept in healthcare, where such emphasis promotes practitioners to not only understand patients' perspectives but to engage with them also.

As previously discussed in earlier chapters, the term EI has often been used interchangeably and has many facets and interpretations. Mayer and Salovey (1997) suggested that EI is:

'the ability to perceive emotions, to access and generate emotions so as to assist thought, to understand emotions and emotional knowledge and reflectively regulate emotions so as to promote emotional and intellectual growth' (Reproduced with permission of Perseus Books Group).

This was further supported by Goleman (1998), who purported that EI ought to be understood in terms of 'the capacity for recognising our own feelings and those of others, for motivating ourselves, and for managing emotions well in ourselves and in our relationships' (p. 317). In consideration of such statements, one could interpret that emotions may be managed and developed, and as such provide a platform for further exploration and discussion later in this chapter. Whilst the factual conceptualisation of EI is a contested subject for discussion, what is less contested is the importance and value of emotionally intelligent individuals within health and social care professions.

EMOTIONAL INTELLIGENCE IN NURSING AND OTHER HEALTHCARE PROFESSIONS

As discussed, EI is the ability to recognise and have an awareness of our emotions and the emotions of others (Goleman 1998). Cadman and Brewer (2001) suggest that there are many attributes and behaviours associated with EI that are congruent with the mission of nursing. EI allows nurses to develop therapeutic relationships (*see* Chapter 4, The therapeutic relationship and EI), care for clients and their families, and manage stress. They state that: 'The ability to empathise, be self-aware, motivate others, have successful relationships, and maintain self-control is an important aspect of professional nursing'. In particular, nursing is a complex profession that requires professional nurses to interact holistically with a variety of individuals in a high-stress environment. Goleman (1998) suggested that EI matters more as the complexity of the work increases, which is congruent in the workforce of nurses. EI includes self-awareness, awareness of others and empathy. Although it is thought that many healthcare employees already possess these skills, research has shown that this is not always the case. EI can be increased through the development of self-awareness, awareness of others and empathy. It is important for nurses to cultivate these skills because the behaviours associated with EI further support the nursing mission by improving health outcomes (Cadmen and Brewer 2001).

Whilst research suggests that EI is innate, it may also be developed. Through the development of EI, healthcare professionals may improve both personally and professionally. Reeves (2005) suggests that the process to develop EI initially begins with self-awareness. This can be a difficult stage, as it requires individuals to immerse themselves into their own emotional state; exploring how they feel about certain situations. Reflection and self-care behaviours such as writing personal reflective journals and reading relevant literature may improve self-awareness. Once self-awareness is achieved, the next phase is to develop an awareness of others. This can be achieved using the same type of techniques in the self-awareness stage; however, in this stage individuals may now begin to recognise emotions and wish to analyse the situation and explore the meaning of the emotion displayed. The final step within the development of EI is empathy. This is an active step using the knowledge developed in the previous stages. Through discipline and effort, an individual can learn to actively listen to others. This type of listening fosters empathy. Whilst working in a positive, caring environment, personal growth in EI can be enhanced (McMullen 2003).

Emotional intelligence and the four-branch ability model

Distinguished in their earlier work, Mayer and Salovey (2004) suggest that many skills and abilities exist within the concept of EI. As such, these skills and abilities have been used to produce the four-branch ability model. This model is composed of the following branches: 1. perceiving emotions, 2. using emotions, 3. understanding emotions, and 4. management of emotions. We shall now explore this model in further detail.

Branch 1: As shown above, Branch 1 reflects perceived emotion and specifically focuses on the ability to recognise emotions in others' facial and postural expressions. This branch primarily focuses on using the non-verbal communication skills that many healthcare professionals use within their roles (Mayer, Salovey and Caruso 2004, p. 3).

Branch 2: This branch acknowledges that facilitation relies on emotions to assist thought process. Theorists of this subject have previously discussed the notion of 'feeling' and the physiological signs of some emotions (Schwarz 1990). It is discussed that a component of intelligence requires a knowledge base that continually develops according to emotional experiences. Such knowledge is believed to facilitate the link between emotion and thought; this is considered valuable in decision-making and planning (Izard 2001).

Branch 3: This branch reflects the understanding of emotion and is noticeably a significant aspect of EI. This branch concentrates on the individual's ability to critically analyse the emotion displayed by others, whilst analysing and appreciating their significance at the time displayed (Mayer, Salovey and Caruso 2004, p. 3).

Branch 4: The fourth branch concludes the branch ability model. It is in this phase that the management of emotion is reflected. It is noticeable that in this branch the personality and attributes of an individual allow for such management to occur (Mayer *et al.* 2004, p. 3).

This model can be brought to bear when looking to exercise emotional labour and the use of emotional touchpoints in clinical practice as a source of learning and development.

Emotional labour

As mentioned earlier another concept associated with EI is that of emotional labour. This was first depicted by Hochschild (1983, p. 7) as 'the induction or suppression of feeling in order to sustain an outward appearance that produces in others a sense of being cared for in a convivial, safe place' (Reproduced with permission of University of California Press-Books).

Huy (1999) consequently made a theoretical connection between emotional labour and EI, suggesting that at specific situations an individual's emotional state may be subject to change if consideration and response is given to such emotions. He also alluded that emotions are a fundamental part of self-adaptation and change. He concluded that EI individuals are able to not only recognise their own and others' emotional states, but also captivate and utilise these emotions to solve problems.

Further theoretical developments of emotional labour over the last decade have widely been discussed. Bolton (2000-01) and Bolton with Boyd (2003) have made important contributions to unravelling the complexity of emotions in healthcare in general and nursing in particular. There has been a great wealth of discussion concerning the cognitive ability to harness the emotional state of professionals within healthcare. Such discussion has alluded that emotionally intelligent professionals use such intelligence to change their cognition and thought process rather than their emotional response in difficult situations (Sakiyama 2011, Fineman 2000-01). Such intelligence as discussed is widely desired by organisations, especially within healthcare, where many professionals are required to deal with difficult emotional situations. This is common within health and social care; there are many publications highlighting the overwhelming emotional strain within many of the professions (Goleman 1998). Within nursing in particular, recent studies have confirmed that the 'emotional labour' contained within the profession requires emotionally intelligent individuals to not only recognise and harness their emotions, but to also work to promote the emotional health of those for whom they care (Cadman and Brewer 2001).

Emotional touchpoints

Whilst there has been an increased interest and discussion pertaining to EI within the platform of health, a new concept that is significantly liked to EI and emotional labour is beginning to emerge. A recent development of growing interest and discussion concerns the importance of patient experience and has been highly publicised as a key aspect in shaping future healthcare services and policies.

Several policies have centralised the 'patient experience' as a national priority within the UK (Darzi 2008, Department of Health 2005). Such development across the UK has seen a trend to place significant importance on the compassionate care delivered within healthcare services. In England, a quality framework has been initiated, following a proposal by Lord Darzi in his report *High Quality Care for All* (Department of Health 2008). This framework uses a scoring mechanism to enable professionals to become mindful of the level of compassionate care they give to their patients. Such a mechanism seeks to educate professionals for what is required to give patients empathetic care. Components of the compassion indicators include smiles, gestures and empathy, all of which encompass the following statement pertaining to emotional labour: 'the induction or suppression of emotions to make others feel safe and cared for' (Hochschild 1983).

The concept of capturing the voices of patients has previously been approached in a number of ways and has focused on exploring attitudes or statements about the positive and negative emotions that have been experienced during a situation, as opposed to specifically focusing on the experience for the individual. Previous research has proved fundamental in this field of interest. Fudge *et al.* (2008) and Bate and Robert (2007) have both highlighted the importance of experiential knowledge from patients as a method to help develop services. Such research has caused further exploration of how this may be developed within health and social care.

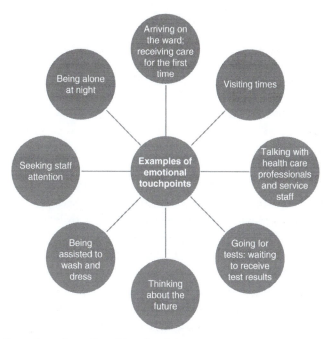

FIGURE 8.1 Examples of emotional touchpoints

Within the NHS Institute for Innovation and Improvement, further development of a number of tools that enable practitioners on the ground to develop more effective services in partnership with patients have recently been initiated. One such method is that of emotional touchpoints. Emotional touchpoints are a tool to help people access their feelings and more readily describe how something felt for them. The method focuses on the specific emotions of patients and their families within key points of the patient journey. During this method, those involved are asked to select from a range of emotional words, those that best describe how they felt about an experience. The method thus helps the interviewer and interviewee to directly focus on the emotion related to the different points (touchpoints) in the patient experience (Dewar *et al.* 2009, pp. 30–1). Such method facilitates professionals in becoming more aware of EI, whilst also developing ways in which they may deliver care using it.

Table 8.1 explores how emotional touchpoints may be used within clinical practice. It is a guideline intended to promote EI.

In addition to developing this approach, Dewar and her colleagues (2010) found that exploring emotional touchpoints with clients helped staff:

- challenge what they thought the client/family wanted
- be more at ease about hearing negative aspects of a client/family experience, as the method doesn't directly focus on blaming the service
- develop better relationships with the client and family members, especially if they had been involved in shaping the service
- take actions going forward that are based on real and meaningful evidence, with staff feeling moved and motivated to have another look at what it is they did.

THE ROLE OF THE REFLECTIVE PRACTITIONER (DRAWING ON EMOTIONAL TOUCHPOINTS)

As previously discussed, Mayer and Salovey (1997) illuminated the possibility that within the concept of EI, professionals have the susceptibility to both develop and change. One particular way in which this development can be facilitated is through reflective practice.

Reflection is the process in which professionals can both conceptualise and achieve better knowledge pertaining to his/her own practice. Various models of reflection currently exist and are used to prompt professionals to question and relive experiences in order to confront, resolve and understand experiences gained through clinical practice (Savage 2003). This could be seen in close comparison to the concept of emotional touchpoints, discussed earlier in this chapter. Whilst the emotional touchpoints tool does educate and also stimulates reflective practice for the professional, it is suggested that to further enhance the professional's EI, a reflective journal using a model for reflection is an effective development strategy.

TABLE 8.1 Emotional touchpoints – a tool to promote EI in both patients and professionals

1	Ask the individual if he/she is happy to discuss with you his/her experiences, and then gain consent.
2	Introduce yourself and the emotional touchpoints tool.
3	Ideally, find a comfortable, confidential place to discuss the individual's experience.
4	Prepare the toolkit; open the case and place the emotion words on one side of the toolkit bag and the event words on the other.
5	Ask the person to pick out or identify the event/s he/she wishes to describe; if the events are not included in the toolkit, ask him/her to describe them.
6	Ask the person to pick out an event that is important to him/her (if the answer is 'none', then write this on a blank card).
7	Ask the person to identify the emotion associated with that event, asking: How did this feel?
8	Try not to rush; give the individual time and space to think and get in contact with those feelings again.
9	This process can be repeated through discussing further events and associated feelings.
10	When you feel as if you have given the person enough time, thank him/her and close the interview.
11	If you feel action is necessary out of the discussions using the touchpoints, you may want to make some agreement that respects confidentiality, boundaries and the interviewed person's safety.
12	Make some notes.
13	Identify areas that were both positive and negative.
14	Consider what changes and or feedback you may need to give to other members of the team.
15	Ask yourself: What can be learned here?
16	Formulate a plan as to what you can do with this information.
17	Consider that the information shared is one person's experience. The reality of the event may be perceived very differently by others, but as you are dealing with a person's feelings, this is how it was for him/her. This demands that we 'try to get into another person's shoes', a cornerstone of dignified care.

(Adapted from Dewar *et al.* 2010)

The following account is taken from this author's own personal reflective journals and depicts how students may use their reflective practice to emulate and develop their personal and professional EI.

Within my second month of placement and within my first year of nurse training, I found myself en route to visit a service user named Ashleigh. My mentor explained to me that she had known Ashleigh for many years and had been involved in many aspects of her care. Ashleigh had cerebral palsy, and as result of this she had many health complications. My mentor went on to explain that Ashleigh until recently had lived in a nursing home for young people with disabilities. She had moved there when her primary care provider, her grandmother, had died. However, Ashleigh had decided that she was now ready to move home and therefore be cared for by agency staff.

On meeting Ashleigh and introducing myself to her, I stood beside her bed. Ashleigh was keen to hold my hand whilst my mentor discussed with her the reason for our visit. Ashleigh agreed to our observation of the procedure, and the carer began preparing the medications as required. Ashleigh kept pulling at my hand, and I had noticed that between her smiles at me she looked as though she was sad. My mentor had noticed this also and could see Ashleigh pulling me closer to her. She began rubbing my hand on her head and crying. My mentor responded and began to talk to Ashleigh about her feelings of being at home again since her grandmother's death. It was very difficult to understand Ashleigh through verbal communication; however, we managed to ascertain through facial expressions, body language and vocalisations that she missed her grandmother and felt alone. Ashleigh soon became inconsolable and was thrashing on her bed. I moved closer and knelt by her bed so that I was able to see her eyes. Without warning Ashleigh pulled me towards her and held me tight. I held her close and tried to sooth her, but I suddenly began to feel overwhelmed with emotion myself. I separated myself from Ashleigh's embrace and tried to collect myself. My feelings were raw and my thoughts were focused on Ashleigh's inability to communicate her grief. My mentor began talking with Ashleigh and her carer about the grieving process. Soon after, Ashleigh began smiling and we were able to supervise the administration of her medicines and schedule further visits for the following days. The following days I continued reflecting on my experience. I had become very emotional at the thought of Ashleigh and the unbearable restriction that her disability caused her in communicating her grief. I could not help but feel immensely frustrated and guilty that both of our experiences of grief were so different, and that for Ashleigh it was determined by her inability to communicate effectively with others.

This experience has since enabled me to learn and develop my understanding of some complex issues surrounding caring for patients that are grieving. It is recognised that some people with disabilities have complex communication needs. A person with complex communication needs may have difficulty expressing his or her emotions, asking questions and conveying information about grief and loss (Scope 2007, p. 30). As in Ashleigh's case, if the person who has died is the primary caregiver, then the loss can be experienced at multiple levels. It is also suggested that persons with a disability may not only experience the loss of someone they care very much about, but potentially they may also experience major changes in their daily routine, living arrangements and financial circumstances. Hence, this loss may also trigger anxiety reactions about their own day-to-day living, care and future (Scope 2007, p. 30).

This experience with Ashleigh has profoundly altered my awareness and desire to explore further and understand how patients with disabilities can both communicate and cope with grief, whilst also exploring how as a student nurse I may learn to become aware of the emotional health of patients. I have found that this experience has not only enabled me to recognise and harness my own emotions, but to also work to promote the emotional health of those I care for.

CONCLUSION

This chapter has been concerned with introducing the new concept of emotional touchpoints as a way of promoting EI. It has explored the relationship between EI, emotional labour and emotional touchpoints. The focus has been to explore how such concepts are currently being developed and used within healthcare, whilst providing some practical tools and examples to assist such development.

REFERENCES

Bate P, Robert G. *Bringing User Experience to Healthcare Improvement: the concepts, methods and practices of experience-based design*. Oxford: Radcliffe Publishing; 2007.

Bolton SC. Who cares? Offering emotion work as a 'gift' in the nursing labour process. *J Adv Nurs*. 2000; **32**(3): 580–6.

Bolton SC, Boyd C. Trolly dolly or skilled emotion manager? Moving on from Hochschild's managed heart. *Work, Employment and Society*. 2003; **17**(2); 289–308.

Cadman C, Brewer J. Emotional intelligence: a vital prerequisite for recruitment in nursing. *J Nurs Manag*. 2001; **9**(6): 321–4.

Cherniss C. Emotional intelligence and the good community. *Am J Community Psychol*. 2002; **30**(1): 1–11.

Darzi A. *High Quality Care for All: NHS Next Stage Review (Final Report)*. London: Department of Health; 2008.

Department of Health. *Now I Feel Tall: what a patient-led NHS feels like*. London: Department of Health; 2005.

Dewar B, Mackay R, Smith S, *et al*. Use of emotional touchpoints as a method of tapping into the experience of receiving compassionate care in a hospital setting. *Journal of Research in Nursing*. 2009; **15**(1): 29–41.

Evans D, Allen H. Emotional Intelligence: its role in training. *Nursing Times*. 2002; **98**(27): 41–2.

Fineman S. *Emotion in Organisations*. London: Sage; 2000.

Fineman S, editor. *The Emotional Organization: passions and power*. Malden, MA: Blackwell Publishing; 2008.

Freshman B, Rubino L. Emotional intelligence: a core competency for health care administrators. *Health Care Manag*. 2002; **20**(4): 1–10.

Freshwater D, Stickley T. The heart of the art: emotional intelligence in nurse education. *Nurs Inq*. 2004; **11**(2): 91–8.

Fudge N, Wolfe CDA, McKevitt C. Assessing the promise of user involvement in health service development: ethnographic study. *BMJ*. 2008; **336**(7639): 313–17.

Goleman D. *Working with Emotional Intelligence*. New York, NY: Bantam; 1998.

Hochschild AR. *The Managed Heart: commercialism of human feeling*. Berkeley, CA: University of California Press; 1983.

Huy QN. Emotional capability, emotional intelligence and radical change. *Acad Manage Rev*. 1999; **24**(2): 325–46.

Izard CE. Emotional intelligence or adaptive emotions? *Journal of Emotion*. 2001; **1**(3): 249–57.

Mayer JD, Salovey P, Caruso D. Competing models of emotional intelligence. In: Sternberg RJ, editor. *Handbook of Human Intelligence*. 2nd ed. New York, NY: Cambridge University Press; 1998.

Mayer JD, Salovey P, Caruso DR. Emotional intelligence: theory, findings, and implications. *Psychological Inquiry*. 2004; **15**: 197–215.

Reeves A. Emotional intelligence: recognizing and regulating emotions. *AAOHN J*. 2005; **53**(4): 172–6.

Sakiyama H. When emotional labour becomes 'good': the use of emotional intelligence. *IJWOE*. 2009; **3**(2): 174–85.

Salovey P, Bedell B, Detweiler JB, *et al*. Coping intelligently: emotional intelligence and the coping process. In: Snyder CR, editor. *Coping: the psychology of what works*. New York, NY: Oxford University Press; 1999. pp. 141–64.

Salovey P, Mayer J. Emotional intelligence. *Imagination, Cognition, and Personality*. 1990; 9(3): 185–211.

Salovey P, Mayer J. What is emotional intelligence? In: Salovey P, Sluyter D, editors. *Emotional Development and Emotional Intelligence: implications for educators*. New York, NY: Basic Books; 1997.

Salovey P, Mayer JD, Goldman SL, *et al*. Emotional attention, clarity, and repair: exploring emotional intelligence using the Trait Meta-Mood Scale. In: Pennebaker JW, editor. *Emotion, Disclosure and Health*. Washington, DC: American Psychological Association; 1995. pp. 125–54.

Salovey P, Woolery A, Mayer JD. Emotional intelligence: conceptualization and measurement. In: Fletcher G, Clark MS, editors. *The Blackwell Handbook of Social Psychology (Vol. 2: Interpersonal Processes)*. Oxford: Blackwell Publishers.

Savage S. Maintaining professional standards. In: Hinchchliff S, Norman S, Schober J, editors. 4th ed. *Nursing Practice and Health Care*. London: Arnold; 2003. pp. 49–75.

Schwarz N. Feelings as information: information and motivational functions of affective states. In: Higgins ET, Sorrentino EM, editors. *Handbook of Motivation and Cognition*. New York, NY: Guilford; 1990. pp. 527–61.

Vitello-Cicciu J. *Leadership Practices and Emotional Intelligence of Nursing Leaders*. Santa Barbara, CA: Fielding Graduate Institute; 2001.

CHAPTER 9

Emotional intelligence and being a successful learner and teacher

Bob Rankin

The pursuit of EI is an important aspect of clinical practice; however, this can only be truly realised with the putting in place of mechanisms to support its uptake. The following two chapters look at approaches and activities that seek to promote and support EI within professional healthcare teaching and education. This chapter looks at the fundamental debate and construct with regards to EI in professional training and education, whilst the subsequent chapter looks at how the use of EI can be fostered and promoted in healthcare professional teaching and education.

INTRODUCTION

It could be argued that for EI to be accepted as a useful construct in education there should be some value attached to defining, measuring, evaluating and applying it. Educators have incorporated a range of manifestations of EI into curricula from preschool through higher education (Humphrey *et al.* 2007), suggesting that the notion of a relationship between EI and the educational process has been generally accepted as valid.

However, this has not been without its controversies, as traditional theorists argue the need for rationality in education (Barchard 2003) and claim that emotions can undermine rational thought. This raises a number of questions for the academic.

- What is the mechanism that links EI with education?
- Does it relate specifically to teaching or learning or both?
- Is EI a trait that we can identify and develop or is it a set of skills that can be taught?

- Is there a clear distinction between EI and IQ, particularly with regard to their impact on academic performance, and if so, how do they differ?
- What are the moral and ethical implications of applying EI theory to education?

Hopefully this chapter will offer some insights on these questions. For clarity, within this chapter, the terms 'learner' and 'helper' will occasionally be used to describe the range of individuals who are relevant to the discussion. The learner could be a pupil, a student, a new member of staff or even an experienced member of staff faced with a new challenge. The 'learner' may also be a patient or client or an individual who is seeking to change his or her perceptions, enhance one's knowledge or modify one's behaviour. The 'helper' may be a teacher, lecturer, mentor, instructor, manager, counsellor, friend or carer. Anyone who is in a helping role may be in a position to foster EI. Of course, this is dependent on EI being an entity that can be developed.

The extent to which EI plays a part in the success of organisations, in particular with regard to learning, will be addressed later in the chapter. To set the context, the mechanism which links EI to learning will be discussed and the evidence base that informs the application of EI in education and in therapeutic interactions will be explored.

THE MECHANISM THAT LINKS EMOTIONAL INTELLIGENCE TO LEARNING

It is difficult to discuss learning without also referring to teaching. Intuitively, we know that, with some exceptions, the quality and style of teaching will impact on the learning process for most individuals. Does emotionally intelligent learning depend on emotionally intelligent teaching, or can it stand alone? The reality is that the relationship between teaching and learning is extremely complex. Teaching can range from facilitation to indoctrination with probably more extreme examples at either end of that spectrum. Learning can be anything from the formation of deeply subconscious associations to forms of higher level learning. Even in the absence of any form of instruction, we still have the capacity to teach ourselves to learn vicariously.

The point is, while we can usually distinguish between the activities of teaching and learning, it is less clear where the boundaries lie within the process. This is especially true when the connection between teaching and learning has an emotional component, a not infrequent occurrence within health and social care education.

There is clear evidence that concentration and memory can be both enhanced and, paradoxically, impaired when emotions are involved (Vos 2006), so the impact of emotion on learning is powerful. During periods of emotional distress, learning is more difficult, yet the salience of an emotion often serves to reinforce learning. The emotionally intelligent teacher will recognise these associations and use emotions to embellish content and challenge learners while recognising the signs and consequences of emotional distress.

APPLYING THEORIES OF EMOTIONAL INTELLIGENCE TO ORGANISATIONS TO ENHANCE LEARNING

In their Best Practice Guidelines to promote EI in the workplace, Goleman *et al.* (1998) proposed that EI can be enhanced by creating an emotionally intelligent environment. More than a decade on, their model continues to provide a useful framework for establishing an organisation which fosters EI. While Goleman and colleagues' model was specifically designed for use in the business world, with the stated intention of improving performance, the model also works in other organisations. Accordingly, an adaptation of this model will be applied to the learning that occurs in academia and in therapeutic environments.

The model describes a process that can be broken into four phases: preparation, training, transfer and maintenance, and finally evaluation, the assumption being that certain conditions can enable individuals to become more emotionally intelligent. The guidelines were collated from an extensive review of supporting research. One of the strong themes throughout this model is the integration of the organisation and the individual. The role of the organisation in promoting EI is reinforced by Kelly *et al.* (2004), who argue that teaching EI will only be successful if it fits in with the ethos of the whole organisation.

Preparation

The preparation phase involves an assessment of the needs and expectations of the organisation as well as an assessment of the individual within it. Without a clear understanding of the strengths and limitations of the organisation, it is difficult to know what it can offer the individual. A therapist with no self-awareness will find it impossible to truly understand the impact that he or she is having on the client, and a teacher with little awareness of his or her subject will struggle to judge the competence of the learner.

Another element of the preparation phase refers to person-centredness. The individual's values and preferences should be considered on the basis that people are better motivated to adapt when they can choose the moment. Student-centredness and client-centredness are well-established principles in education, and therapy and clichés such as 'the customer knows best' indicate that the business world accepts this principle too.

Training

The phase that Goleman *et al.* (1998) refer to as 'training' would also cover activities such as: teaching, working with, educating, instructing, and facilitating, as well as other helping strategies that fit into education and therapeutic interventions. This phase highlights the qualities of the 'trainer', which will enable him or her to reach out and work with the learner. Qualities such as empathy, warmth and genuineness are recognised as important characteristics when engaging with learners. These humanistic qualities underpin many therapeutic relationships, and learners who recognise such qualities in their teachers claim to benefit the most from the learning process (Sava 2002).

Another key element of the 'training' phase involves the ability of the teacher to provide opportunities for learning that are manageable but challenging and to offer feedback which increases insight and growth. Self-awareness is often referred to as the cornerstone of emotional and social intelligence, and this is best achieved by using experiential methods. Teachers and therapists recognise the impact that good feedback can have on the individual's development and consequent future performance and behaviour. Formative learning is greatly enhanced by accurate and constructive feedback. Mistakes are viewed as learning opportunities, and the environment should be able to accommodate genuine mistakes from which learners grow.

Transfer and maintenance

Transfer of learning requires encouragement and reinforcement by the helper. Prompts, cues and role modelling can be invaluable at this stage. The best prompts and cues are those that resonate with the learner and provoke an emotional response that can jolt the senses. Contextual restraints need to be recognised and either overcome or removed to enable progress. The culture within the organisation must be able to support learning. Safety and support will facilitate a positive change, which will be more enduring.

Evaluation

One way of assessing the effectiveness of the organisation in promoting EI is to evaluate it for signs of lasting effect. Baseline indicators can help to highlight areas that have improved, and regular evaluation can help to reduce complacency and maintain developments. Therapists will help their clients to identify early signs of relapse, and this can empower the client to take action where necessary. Ideally, the learning that has occurred during therapy will be applied to novel situations in the future, reaffirming the value of the learning that has been achieved. Educationalists strive for their students to become 'lifelong' learners, as this suggests that the learning process under their tutelage has been accommodated and then assimilated by the learner. To a certain extent, their job is done!

Box 9.1 Social-based activity

With a peer, review the learning and teaching you have been receiving and giving in light of the approach outlined above. Identify areas where this learning and teaching is using and/or enhancing EI.

Now identify areas where the learning and teaching you have been receiving and giving is an 'EI-free zone'. Core questions to consider include the following.
- What learning outcomes have no relevance to EI, if any?
- What barriers are there to implementing a more EI-focused approach?
- Are some environments better suited than others to incorporate EI, and why?

The process described above suggests that it is possible to apply a model of EI to learning and teaching by creating an environment which integrates the processes of education for the learner and for the helper. The emotionally intelligent helper can recognise the role of emotions in learning and will also be aware of the negative impact of emotional distress. Therefore, learning that is enquiry-based or experiential provides the helper with the opportunity to include emotional cues to enhance understanding. The true test of EI in the helper will be whether he or she recognises signs of distress in the learner resulting from inappropriate expectations or personal stressors provoked by the learning process.

TRAIT EMOTIONAL INTELLIGENCE VERSUS ABILITY EMOTIONAL INTELLIGENCE

To a certain extent, the relationship between EI and learning needs to defined within the discussion that surrounds trait and ability EI. In order to truly establish the extent to which EI can be learned, it is essential to be able to accurately measure baseline and acquired levels of EI. Therefore, is it appropriate to consider EI in terms of an individual trait, or should we view it as a set of skills that can be applied?

Ascribing 'trait EI' to an individual implies that it is a quality or a characteristic, rather like a personality trait, which will determine, to an extent, how that individual behaves in any given situation. Whether this particular trait comes from inherent components of the person or develops through exposure is less important to this discussion than the premise that it exists in a form that can be subjectively identified by the person and/or objectively identified by others. In other words, the person may be able to convey this trait by their responses to a self-report tool, or it could be that others may reflect the trait in a reference or an appraisal or make an informal judgment of the individual. In either case, the EI that is being identified is accepted as a component of the individual's personality, clarified over time, which potentially drives their behaviour. Essentially, according to this model, the individual possesses EI.

To distinguish between the ability model and the trait model of EI, Petrides and Furnham (2001) and Petrides (2009) refer to trait as 'self concept' and 'perceived ability' rather than actual ability. Trait EI is sometimes referred to as 'trait emotional self-efficacy'. While traits can be perceived and acknowledged by the individual, they can also be ascribed by others. To an extent, an employment referee draws on trait theory when providing a profile of the individual's qualities and characteristics while judging suitability for a job, which is presumed to be objectively based on previous performance. The assumption is that there is an accurate, predictive relationship between the assessment of traits such as EI and future performance. This tends to disregard, or at least minimise, the confounding impact of: context, occupational roles, new expectations, the environment, colleagues and a whole raft of other factors that can influence future performance. Accordingly, the reliability of such an assessment is called into question. Self-reports are also regarded with similar reservations; it could be argued that the individual's self-concept can only truly be tested for accuracy in light of the individual's subsequent behaviour. Furthermore, one's behaviour and success or otherwise in a job will impact on one's future self-concept.

In contrast with 'trait EI', a judgment of 'ability EI' requires the individual to perform prescribed tasks to a predetermined standard to enable an evaluation of performance. The assumption is that EI is something that can be demonstrated through competencies. That is, we should be measuring what people actually do rather than what they or others believe they *will* do. It may be argued that EI is of little value unless it can be demonstrated by actions that can be objectively assessed, and measures of 'ability' EI claim to do just that.

The most commonly applied test that is used to measure ability EI is the Mayer–Salovey–Caruso Emotional Intelligence Test (MSCEIT) (Mayer *et al.* 2002). This is based on an IQ-style ability test that examines the person's abilities on each of the four components of EI outlined in Chapter 1.

Bradberry and Su (2003) criticised the MSCEIT, claiming that it lacked face validity and predictive validity in the workplace. One of the main concerns is that it is modelled on IQ tests, yet the answers are not objectively defined. There is also an issue in that It would be impossible for respondents to arrive at novel and insightful conclusions with regard to EI since the 'norm' would always be viewed as the best response.

Box 9.2   Reflective activity

Consider and reflect on the following:
- if learning or teaching others to become emotionally intelligent means conformity rather than originality, what are the positive advantages?
- what are the implications if the consensus opinion is always correct, particularly when emotion is involved?

Within the context of the clear limitations of trait and ability EI, mixed models have evolved. Goleman's model of EI (Goleman 1998) introduces four main components: self-awareness, self-management, social awareness and relationship management.

Goleman includes competencies within this framework, which he claims are not so much innate abilities as capabilities that need opportunities to be developed. Goleman has received strong criticism of his model, with accusations in some quarters that it lacks scientific rigour and that, in trying to encompass all perspectives, it panders to populist notions of EI (Mayer *et al.* 2008). Locke (2005) characterises mixed models as being 'preposterously all encompassing' (Locke 2005, p. 428). However, Goleman's four-factor construct of EI has been incorporated into assessment tools that have been acknowledged as fundamental to the conceptualisation of EI.

The premise that self reports are able to measure self-efficacy, and that ability tests can objectively measure performance, would suggest that there is merit in a study which correlated self reports with measures of ability. Kirk *et al.* (2009) found a significant correlation between a self report, which measured self-efficacy, and scores on the MSCEIT. Perhaps it is the distinction between trait and ability EI rather than the similarities that may provide the key to achieving better reliability and validity in the field of EI research.

While trait and ability tests both measure different facets of EI, as with all human behavioural research, the goal should be to identify antecedents and attempt to relate these to outcomes. Perhaps matching traits to behaviour could help to clarify the elements of EI that might truly make a difference. Once the distinctions between trait EI and ability EI are fully established, the mechanism that links them may well become much more significant to researchers than the differences. It is also likely that trait and ability EI are not mutually exclusive; therefore, exploring their complementary dimensions and analysing any predictive relationships will undoubtedly be an area for future research. If it was possible to demonstrate a reliable predictive relationship between trait and ability measures of EI, it would be reasonable to conclude that an individual who possesses EI will perform in an emotionally intelligent manner.

It is important to be able to identify both trait and ability elements of EI on the basis that emotionally intelligent behaviour requires a source. If trait EI can be linked to better outcomes in education, there is clear merit in being able to identify and assess the trait, its consequent behaviour and the relationship between the two.

EMOTIONAL INTELLIGENCE VERSUS IQ

Traditional measures of intelligence have been used to predict success in learning for almost 100 years. The premise of this is that an objective measure of intelligence (IQ) will provide the best evidence of learning potential. An assertion that EI is a better predictor of success than IQ (Goleman 2005) challenges this notion. However, what evidence currently exists that enables us to scientifically distinguish between IQ and EI? How can we be sure that measures of EI are not simply replicating measures of general intelligence, or 'g'?

The only real justification for developing and applying measures of EI would be that they measure criteria that are clearly distinct from 'g', otherwise the IQ test would suffice. Since its early applications, the predictability of measures of IQ has been widely accepted. However, Wechsler (1940) defined intelligence as: 'the aggregate or global capacity of the individual to act purposefully, to think rationally and to deal effectively with his environment' (p. 444). In referring to 'non-intellective' elements of intelligence such as affective, personal and social factors, Wechsler claimed that these elements were essential for success in life. Cognitive ability on its own, without the non-intellective elements, would not be enough to cope with interpersonal and intrapersonal challenges. Hunter and Hunter (1984) concurred with Wechsler and claimed that IQ accounts for less than 25% of variance in predicting job performance, suggesting that some other ingredient, over and above 'g', must be present.

Mayer *et al.* (2004) suggest the EI is a discriminant construct from IQ and go on to make a number of claims to differentiate the two. Mayer *et al.* (2004) clearly identify EI as a measurable ability and highlight through their work that it can be distinguished from other measurable constructs such as personality and intelligence. Key points of difference between EI and these other constructs include that those people with highter EI have healthier interpersonal realtionships and consequently have more extensive and better quality social supports than those with lower EI measures. Additionally, people with higher EI are less likely to misuse alcohol or drugs.

Mayer *et al.* (2004) also claim that there is no evidence to demonstrate that the behaviours highlighted above correlate with measures of IQ, which suggests that measures of EI, while still developing, are measuring something other than IQ. There are certainly potential advantages of being able to clearly distinguish between EI and IQ: 'One of the factors that contribute to the popularity of EI is the belief in the possibility that, unlike IQ, EI may be improved. There is a sense that this might be a refreshing break from the apparently "fixed" quality of IQ' (Rankin 2009, p. 42).

The notion that EI can be developed is not universally accepted with strong argument being forwarded through the construct of personality. McCrae (2000) in particular suggests that personality traits are more influential upon behaviour than EI. These personality traits have been explored in depth over many years and are consistently found to be quite fixed throughtout adulthood. McCrae (2000) forwards that given this it seems overly optimistic to suggest that components of EI can be altered within adults.

The apparent positive correlation between age and EI (Bar-On 2000) would appear to support the assertion that it can, indeed, be enhanced. It certainly cannot be claimed that EI is fixed when older individuals score higher than younger individuals. It appears as though nature and nurture combine to enable the individual's capacity to be achieved in the field of EI, which is typical in most areas of cognitive development.

There is a wide consensus that general intelligence, 'g', is stable. During our early years, 'Piagetian' stages of cognitive development occur. This involves the assimilation of new knowledge into existing levels of understanding, which is then followed by accommodation, whereby the individual adjusts his or her understanding and knowledge in the face of new information (Santrock 2008). Stage-like developments of cognitive ability such as these are more obvious in children but become less obvious with age. New insights and sudden changes in perspective can accompany moments of discovery, regardless of age, suggesting that knowledge and reasoning may continue to be enhanced. This does not necessarily imply that intelligence has increased. Our general intelligence, as measured by IQ, determines the limits of our potential.

Applying the same analogy to EI, this may be a potential capacity for using and understanding emotions. This potential can only be met through exposure to and increasing awareness of emotions. 'One could argue that we all have a unique potential to achieve our own level of EI and, for this potential to be realised, we require the necessary experiences. Without the correct opportunities, it would be difficult for any of us to reach our potential. Perhaps "potential emotional intelligence" is best described as "trait", whereas the extent to which this potential is being met is best described as "ability"' (Rankin 2009, p. 44).

Liptak (2005) promotes five steps to enhancing EI competencies for the learner: help the learner to recognise the importance of EI skills; identify the learner's EI skill deficits; assess the learner's EI strengths; help the learner to explore barriers to being successful in the workplace and then practise the relevant skills.

EMOTIONAL INTELLIGENCE AND ETHICAL VALUES

Emerling and Goleman (2003) raise the controversial question about whether individuals who are higher in EI will automatically possess higher moral standards. To what extent, therefore, are morals and values related to EI and learning? It is expected that psychological research will apply a value-neutral approach; however, there is a general inference that the traits associated with EI are intrinsically linked to positive behaviour towards others.

There is no guarantee that EI would necessarily be used by the 'helper' for altruistic purposes, and if the helper is skilled in recognising and managing the emotions of the learner, is it conceivable that this skill might be used for the manipulation of others? Gardner (1999) claims that intelligence is neither moral nor immoral, citing the persuasive skills of Nazi leaders and great comedians who could deftly manipulate the emotions of crowds. There is an expectation that manipulative individuals will have diminished empathic abilities; this does not fit comfortably with models of EI – one of the many attractions of EI is the orientation towards others. This tends to support the notion that EI is more likely to be used as a positive trait rather than a negative one.

THE RELATIONSHIP BETWEEN EMOTIONAL INTELLIGENCE AND SUCCESSFUL LEARNING

In a study of the impact of EI on the attainment of nursing students, a significant predictive relationship was found between students' EI scores, using Schutte and colleagues' Assessing Emotions Scale (2007), and subsequent success in academic performance (Rankin 2009). Indeed, the relationship between EI and academic performance was stronger than the relationship between entrance qualifications and academic performance. While prior academic attainment remains the traditional method used by higher education institutions to predict the performance of students, the relationship between EI and academic success appears to be more powerful. When the effects of other antecedents, such as age, gender and prior academic attainment, are controlled, the predictive relationship between EI and other programme outcomes, such as practice performance and attrition, is also significant. The correlation between EI and practice performance is of particular importance with regard to recruitment and selection in nurse education. The relationship between EI and successful learning is discussed more fully in Chapter 10.

CONCLUSION

There appears to be enough evidence to suggest that EI is a central factor for successful learning on health and social care courses. The relationship may indicate a stronger potential overall for learning among students with higher levels of EI, or it may simply be that EI is a quality that fits well with the expectations of health and social care education and is, therefore, readily recognised by mentors.

Without comparing baseline EI with measures of EI at the end of an educational programme, it is not possible to ascertain whether EI has indeed been developed. Empirical studies have been accused of trying to measure changes in EI by retrospectively looking at vaguely related qualities (Humphrey et al. 2007). Ideally, research should be comparing 'like with like'. However, there is sufficient evidence to suggest that EI can be taught (Bar-On 2000), that EI enhances learning (Rankin 2009), and that the means to achieve these ends have been offered within this chapter.

REFERENCES

Barchard KA. Does emotional intelligence assist in the prediction of academic success? *Educational and Psychological Measurement.* 2003; **63**(5): 840–58.

Bar-On R. In: Parker JDA, editor. *The Handbook of Emotional Intelligence.* San Francisco, CA: Jossey-Bass; 1999.

Bradberry T, Su L. Ability versus skill-based assessment of emotional intelligence. *Psicothema.* 2003; **18**(Suppl.): 59–66.

Emmerling RJ, Goleman D. Emotional intelligence: issues and common misunderstandings. *Issues and Recent Developments in Emotional Intelligence.* 2003; available at: www.eiconsortium.org

Gardner H. Who owns intelligence? *The Atlantic Monthly.* 1999; **283**(2): 67–76.

Goleman D. *Working with Emotional Intelligence.* London: Bloomsbury Publishing; 1998.

Goleman D. *Emotional Intelligence: why it matters more than IQ.* 10th anniversary ed. New York, NY: Bantam Dell; 2005.

Humphrey N, Curran A, Morris E, *et al.* Emotional intelligence and education: a critical review. *Educational Psychology.* 2007; **27**(2): 235–54.

Hunter JE, Hunter RF. Validity and utility of alternative predictors of job performance. *Psychological Bulletin*. 1984; **96**(1): 72–98.

Kelly B, Longbottom J, Potts F, *et al.* Applying emotional intelligence: exploring the PATHS curriculum. *Educational Psychology in Practice*. 2004; **20**: 221–40.

Kirk BA, Schutte NS, Hine DW. Development and preliminary validation of an emotional self-efficacy scale. *Personality and Individual Differences*. 2009; **45**(6): 432–6.

Liptak JJ. Using emotional intelligence to help students succeed in the workplace. *Journal of Employment Counselling*. 2005; **42**: 172–80.

Locke EA. Why emotional intelligence is an invalid concept. *Journal of Organizational Behavior*. 2005; **26**(4): 425–31.

Mayer JD, Roberts R, Barsade SG. Human abilities: emotional intelligence. *Annual Review of Psychology*. 2008; **59**: 507–36.

Mayer JD, Salovey P. The intelligence of emotional intelligence. *Intelligence*. 1993; **17**(4): 433–42.

Mayer JD, Salovey P, Caruso D. *Mayer-Salovey-Caruso Emotional Intelligence Test (MSCEIT) User's Manual*. Toronto: MSH; 2002.

Mayer JD, Salovey P, Caruso DR. A further consideration of the issues of emotional intelligence. *Psychological Enquiry*. 2004; **15**: 249–55.

McCrae RR. Emotional intelligence from the perspective of the Five-Factor Model. In: Bar-On R, Parker JDA, editors. *The Handbook of Emotional Intelligence*. Jossey-Bass, San Francisco; 2000.

Petrides KV. *Technical Manual for the Trait Emotional Intelligence Questionnaires (TEIQue)*. London: London Psychometric Laboratory; 2009.

Petrides KV, Furnham A. Trait Emotional intelligence: psychometric investigation with reference to established trait taxonomies. *European Journal of Personality*. 2001; **15**: 425–48.

Rankin RF. *Emotional Intelligence: attrition and attainment in nursing and midwifery education* [doctoral thesis]. Available at: http://hdl.handle.net/1893/2321 (accessed 17 July 2011).

Santrock JW. *A Topical Approach to Life Span Development*. New York, NY: McGraw-Hill; 2008.

Sava FA. Causes and effects of teacher conflict-inducing attitudes towards pupils: a path analysis model. *Teaching and Teacher Education*. 2002; **18**: 1007–21.

Schutte NS, Malouff JM, Bhullar N. In: Stough C, Saklofske D, Parker J, editors. *The Assessment of Emotional Intelligence*. Springer Publishing.

Vos J. *The New Learning Revolution*. UK: Network Press; 2006.

Wechsler D. Non-intellective factors in general intelligence. *Psychological Bulletin*. 1940; **37**: 444–5.

CHAPTER 10

Educational approaches and activities to enhance emotional intelligence

Kim Foster and Heather McKenzie

'*An education that ignores the value and development of the emotions is one that denies the very heart of the art of [nursing] practice. By focusing entirely on the rational, we are in danger of producing unbalanced practitioners. When teachers pay little or no attention to emotional development, they fail to communicate with students the significance of human relationships.*' (Freshwater and Stickley 2004, p. 93, reproduced with permission of John Wiley and Sons)

Freshwater and Stickley (2004) make a compelling call for education that facilitates learning about the 'messy' business of human relations – with the 'self' as well as with patients and colleagues. Theoretical knowledge and development of technical or clinical skills are only some of the requisite abilities for nurses, doctors and other health and social care professionals. Consistent with the recognised need to strengthen EI educational preparation in the health and social care professions, this chapter explores educational learning theories and practical classroom and clinical activities that aim to enhance health and social care professionals' EI. We have focused on applying theory to the practice of learning and teaching emotional intelligence with the premise that EI is not necessarily inherent and can be learned and improved. We believe everyone can be assisted to develop their emotional literacy.

This chapter concentrates on educational approaches that enhance EI, and the discussion and activities are equally relevant for health and social care students and practitioners. As discussed in Chapter 1, there are a number of theoretical models and definitions of EI and the construct itself is open to debate. In this chapter we have taken a broad approach to EI, and, consistent with Hurley (2008), discuss EI in terms of an intelligence that includes self-awareness and self-management, communication, collaboration and relatedness, and an ability to show empathy and develop reflexivity.

APPROACHES TO EMOTIONAL INTELLIGENCE EDUCATION AND TRAINING

The literature on adult education for EI, particularly in the health and social care professions, includes a range of approaches to education and training. These can be grouped into two broad categories – undergraduate or preregistration education and curriculum that includes clinical education; and work-based training programs for practising health professionals. We outline approaches relevant for both groups, with a focus on undergraduate educational approaches.

Preparing for emotional intelligence education

Cherniss *et al.* (1998), in a thorough review of research and literature on EI education and training, propose guidelines for developing programs to strengthen EI. Their review focused on workplace training; however, the principles are also relevant for undergraduate curricula. Table 10.1 summarises the guidelines in four phases of educational development. These form a useful framework for educators

TABLE 10.1 Guidelines for best practice in educating for EI

1 Paving the way for change	**2 Doing the work of change**
• Assess needs of organisation for most critical competencies	• Foster a positive educator/learner relationship
• Assess needs of individual for competencies needed for his/her practice	• Make learning self-directed
• Assess with care and include feedback on strengths and weaknesses	• Set clear goals for specific behaviours and skills
• Maximise learners' choices so as to facilitate motivation to change	• Break goals into manageable steps
• Encourage stakeholders' participation	• Provide opportunity to practice
• Link learning goals to personal values	• Provide feedback on performance
• Build positive expectations	• Focus on experiential methods
• Assess readiness for education and training	• Include support mechanisms
	• Use role models (live or audiovisual)
	• Strengthen insight and self-awareness
	• Prevent relapse
3 Encouraging transfer and maintenance of change	**4 Evaluating change**
• Encourage use of skills on the job using mentoring and/or coaching	• Evaluate change in competence or skills using appropriate measures
• Develop an organisational culture that supports learning	• Evaluate before and after training and follow up if possible

(Adapted from Cherniss *et al.* 1998)

who are developing EI programs. Cherniss *et al.* (1998) make a number of points with regard to the guidelines:

- each phase is important in its own right but closely interrelates with the others
- the phases are (and therefore EI educational approaches need to be) additive and incremental, starting with preparation and moving through training to evaluation
- while learning experiences do not necessarily need to adhere to all of the guidelines, success is likely to increase with each one that is followed.

In particular, Cherniss *et al.* (1998) note the need for evaluation of these educational programs and approaches. As Clarke (2006) cautions, while there may be numerous programs aimed at developing EI, there is limited research into the impact this education can have on individuals' EI capacity. In the authors' experience, part of the challenge of educating for EI is to demonstrate evidence for the efficacy and outcomes of the work. Educators who are considering developing and implementing EI theory and education into undergraduate curricula or workplace training also need to consider embedding evaluation strategies into their educational plan from the outset.

Educating for EI necessarily involves a process of change and development in the learner and in his or her attitudes towards, and relationships with, self and others (Cherniss *et al.* 1998). In aiming to effect change in learners, and consistent with self-management as integral to EI, educators need to be prepared to identify and manage their own emotional abilities. Role modelling is an integral feature of successful EI education (Cadman and Brewer 2001, Freshwater and Stickley 2004) and as such requires educators to be self-aware and address their own understandings and abilities for this work. This is perhaps one of the more challenging aspects of EI education!

Table 10.2 outlines some questions educators may find useful as they prepare to deliver education on EI. Educators may also consider engaging in formal or informal debriefing and/or focused conversations with experienced professional colleagues, e.g. in clinical supervision. The need for reflexivity (discussed later) is as important for educators as it is for learners.

A further issue to consider when developing EI educational programs is the mode of delivery. The delivery of programs depends on the availability of human and financial resources (including appropriately trained educators); the relative priority given to EI within an overall program of health and social care education; and geographical and time constraints for learners and educators. The most appropriate mode of delivery for EI education is a matter of debate, with persuasive arguments for and against face-to-face delivery as opposed to online or distance education. Hurley (2008), for example, indicates there is evidence that communication and socialisation, as integral components of learning EI, can be effectively developed through web-based education and that online or distance education may offer a

TABLE 10.2 Reflecting on self – some questions for EI educators and trainers

- Do I recognise and manage my emotions effectively?
- Do I know my strengths and limitations?
- Do I show interest in and concern for others?
- Am I a good listener?
- Am I dependable and trustworthy?
- Am I comfortable with new ideas? Am I willing to persist despite challenges and setbacks?
- Do I take responsibility for my own performance?

Adapted from Bellack (1999, p. 4)

viable addition or alternative to face-to-face EI education. Cadman and Brewer (2001), however, argue that the abilities associated with EI are best learnt through close learner/educator relationships. Cherniss (2000) contends that the role of the educator and the relationship between him/her and the learner is crucial in providing a safe and supportive learning environment in which learners can develop their EI ability. The authors' own view is that while these abilities may be developed through online education, they are most effectively developed through face-to-face contact. Nonetheless, online information, discussion and activities, and online audiovisual materials such as videos demonstrating communication and interaction can be very effective tools and supplements to face-to-face learning.

Learning theories for emotional intelligence education

As with other undergraduate and work-based education programs, EI education is underpinned by principles of lifelong learning and adult learning. These are strongly relevant to EI education, as the abilities we aim to develop with learners will be honed over time and with incremental learning opportunities.

Adult learning theories have significantly influenced the development of education programs for healthcare professionals. The work of Knowles (1984) in particular has contributed to an increasing focus on experiential, problem-focused learning in which students take some responsibility for setting their own learning agendas and educators use an andragogical, rather than pedagogical, approach to working with students. In essence, this includes students and educators working closely together in a relationship that is less hierarchical than more traditional pedagogical learning relationships, and the recognition that adults are likely to have specific learning styles and motivations. The concept of self-directed learning is closely associated with Knowles' andragogy theory. This adult learning approach, which encourages students to set their own learning goals and outcomes, has been widely used in healthcare (Levett-Jones, 2005). In this chapter, we focus on two particular adult learning theories that have been used to inform EI education in the healthcare professions. These are transformative learning theory and social learning theory.

Transformative learning and teaching

Transformative learning is an educational theory of adult learning by Mezirow (1997, 2000) that refers to a process of creating change in learners' *frames of reference*. Frames of reference help us to make sense of the world in which we live and can be seen as having two dimensions:

- **habits of mind:** abstract, broad and habitual ways of thinking, feeling, and acting, e.g. ethnocentrism – viewing others outside our own group as being inferior
- **point of view**: resulting feelings, beliefs and judgments we have about specific people or groups that are subject to alteration as our assumptions change, e.g. attitudes towards welfare recipients.

Transformative learning aims to develop *autonomous thinking* through critical reflection on the assumptions through which our beliefs, habits of mind or points of view are based. Thus, *transformations* in frames of reference (such as ethnocentrism) can take place. Mezirow (1997) argues that transformative learning is based in the way we communicate, and in order to facilitate transformative learning, educators need to help learners become aware of, and critical about, their own and others' assumptions. Learning takes place through discovery, and learning activities include critical incidents, role plays, case studies, simulated experiences, analysis of metaphors, consciousness raising, group projects and learning contracts. According to Mezirow (1997), transformative learning can be considered the essence of adult education.

Teaching for transformative learning is therefore learner-centred, participatory and involves group problem-solving. In this process, educators become facilitators and *provocateurs* rather than subject authorities (Mezirow, 1997). Teaching moves away from the didactic to a facilitated dialogue and interaction between learner and educator. Principles of transformative teaching include building a critical consciousness in learners and thinking critically, and forming a student–teacher relationship as a partnership where there is opportunity for dialogue and students are encouraged to voice their opinions on issues, to appreciate differences, and to build a sense of community (McAllister 2005). A transformative learning environment can support learners to be critically reflective and self-determining, and it can strengthen their capacity to confidently address issues and challenges they may encounter in the health and social care environment (Foster *et al.* 2009).

Health and social care educational programs and curricula that have EI at the core, offered within a transformative learning and teaching environment, provide an opportunity for education to revolutionise learners and their practice (Freshwater and Stickley 2004). In this way, the process of transformation in EI education can be considered circular and interdependent. While transformative learning theory can provide a pedagogical foundation from which to develop EI in learners, Mezirow (2000) argues that participation in transformative learning itself requires that the learner have emotional 'maturity' or intelligence.

Social learning theory

For education of health professionals to be transformative (Mennin 2010), deep engagement of students with the complex realities of human life is critical. In this regard, social learning theories can inform EI educational initiatives in important ways. As Bleakley points out, social learning theories:

'stress the importance of both context (learning is situated) and process (learning is dynamic) ... [They] focus on processes of collaboration, means of access to distributed knowledge, how knowledge acquires legitimacy and meaning, knowledge production rather than reproduction, socialisation as a process of learning and identity construction as a learning outcome' (2010, p. 851, reproduced with permission of John Wiley and Sons).

First developed by Bandura (1977) in the 1970s, social learning theory provides a framework for understanding learning as a social process in which there is a dynamic relationship between the environment or context and the interactions embedded within it. We argue here that this framework facilitates engagement with the complexity that is inherent in healthcare settings and, most particularly, in relationships within healthcare settings. Health professional students are exposed to that complexity early in their education programs. It is therefore critical that educators focus on strengthening their abilities to manage and engage with complex situations and relationships, all of which inevitably involve emotionality.

This way of approaching health professional education for EI can facilitate deep learning that is meaningful in that it both recognises the 'self' that the student brings to a situated learning activity, and also the intersubjective connections that will flow from a situation in which one person is responsive to another's misfortune. Clarke's work (2010) is particularly interesting in this regard. He argues that EI can be enhanced through team-based, situated learning experiences and that the intensity of team engagement can have an impact on the development of some aspects of EI. Clarke suggests that it is the relational ties and bonds that develop within teams engaged in activities involving the sharing of emotional knowledge that can have the greatest effects on improving EI. This is important for our understanding of the benefits of situated, team-based, social learning in health professional education programs. Healthcare settings frequently demand the foregrounding of emotionality and the sharing of emotional knowledge; engaging students in team-based learning activities that facilitate their understandings of this and their confidence in working with emotions, both their own and those of others, is fundamental to the development of their professional identity and confidence.

Educating for emotional intelligence

While there is inconsistency in the literature as to the EI components that should be included in health professional undergraduate/pre-registration curricula and/or workplace programs, there are a number of common intrapersonal and interpersonal

TABLE 10.3 Elements of an emotionally intelligent curriculum

- Reflective learning experiences
- Role modelling
- Supportive supervision and mentoring
- Inclusion of the arts and humanities in learning/teaching
- Focus on developing 'self' and relationships
- Focus on developing empathy
- Commitment to emotional literacy and competency

Adapted from Freshwater and Stickley (2004, p. 96)

elements. These include the development of: *self-awareness* (McQueen 2004, Hurley 2008), *empathy* (Freshwater and Stickley 2004, Grewal and Davidson 2008, Hurley 2008, Roberts 2010, Stratton *et al.* 2008) and *interpersonal and communication skills* (Grewal and Davidson 2008; Stratton, Saunders and Elam 2008). In accordance with our view of EI as construct (at the beginning of the chapter), in this section we discuss approaches and strategies that can be used to develop these particular aspects of EI. As seen in the following discussion, while we have addressed them separately, there is considerable overlap between them. The educational activities discussed under each EI component are often applicable to the other components, and as noted earlier, the combination of activities and the incremental development of EI abilities is important when educating and training for EI. *See* Table 10.3 for an outline of the elements of an emotionally intelligent curriculum.

Strengthening self-awareness

Self-awareness is considered the cornerstone of EI (Cherniss *et al.* 1998) and includes knowing our values, biases and attitudes towards others and situations, and how we are likely to respond in particular circumstances. Self-awareness also involves knowing how our needs might impact on our work as health professionals (Jackson and O'Brien 2009). In being aware of our own emotional and personal characteristics, abilities, strengths and vulnerabilities – in other words, our intrapersonal elements – health and social care professionals have a basis from which they can address, modify, manage and/or strengthen these aspects of the 'self' in their work.

Arguably, without knowing one's 'self' it is difficult to understand the 'other', and, indeed, to work interpersonally and relate effectively to others in a professional capacity. Hurley (2008), for example, identifies that in reviews of professional practice in nursing the enhancement of self-awareness is considered pivotal in educational preparation for the discipline, particularly in mental health, where the use of self is a key component of therapeutic practice. The health professional's exploration of 'self' is therefore commonly considered a fundamental place from which to commence practice. Being self-aware and able to attend to our own feelings and experiences contributes to the therapeutic use of self with patients and families (Foster,

McAllister and O'Brien 2006), and, in order to interact effectively with patients and families, practitioners first need to be able to differentiate and understand their own experience as separate from others (Gallop and O'Brien 2003).

In being self-aware and attuned to the differences between self and others, health and social care practitioners often engage in reflective practice. Reflection in relation to practice is a core component of most undergraduate education for health and social care practitioners, as it provides an avenue to critically consider personal values and behaviours, and to use the resulting insights to strengthen their work. This process becomes even more crucial once practitioners enter the workforce (Usher, Foster and Stewart 2008). Processes such as reflective journaling are often used to encourage learners to develop their self-awareness, and more recently this process has been specifically applied to strengthening emotional competence. Harrison and Fopma-Loy (2010), for example, found that progressive, reflective journal prompts could be useful tools to stimulate learners' reflection on aspects of EI. Clinical supervision is another avenue for practitioners to engage in self-awareness. Clinical supervision is a process where practitioners' clinical work and their interactions with patients and families is the focus of reflection with another experienced clinician (Jackson and O'Brien 2009). It is a formal and structured way to learn and reflect on actions within the context of a supportive relationship and can involve either individual or group supervision. Clinical supervision is therefore one of a number of ways in which practitioners engage in reflective practice and strengthen their self-awareness (Clouder and Sellars 2004).

Self-awareness learning activities

Self-awareness is a core component of health and social care education and training, with a range of activities commonly used to encourage greater awareness of 'self' characteristics. The 'Johari Window', for example, is a frequently used tool for developing self-awareness. The Johari Window is a model involving four aspects of self. These include aspects that are *known* to self, and/or *known* to others; aspects that are *unknown* to others (but may be *known* to self), and aspects *unknown* to self that are may be either *known* or *unknown* to others. These are often configured in a diagram with four quadrants or sections. The aim is to expand self-awareness, i.e. the quadrant *known* to self – and reduce those aspects that are *unknown* to self and *unknown* to others (Luft 1969).

There are a number of ways in which the 'Window' has been used to encourage self-reflection and awareness. One common activity that the authors of this chapter have used is to pair students up, then give them a sheet with a blank Johari Window divided into four quadrants and a separate list of adjectives describing various individual characteristics or qualities, most of which are positive in tone, e.g. 'kind', 'active', 'serene'. Students are asked to identify the five adjectives they consider best describe them, and transfer these to the quadrant 'known to self'. They are then asked to choose around five or so adjectives they consider best describe the other student, and to share these with their partner. Students then transfer these adjectives to the respective quadrants (either *'known* to self' if they are the same as the ones they have chosen for themselves, or *'not* known to self'). Student pairs discuss the insights they have gained with each other, and then larger group discussion can address broader issues of how self-understanding can strengthen health and social care practice. In the authors' experience, the exercise is informative and often affirming for students, as they gain insight about themselves through the feedback from their peers.

Reflective learning activities – using the arts and humanities

Consistent with Freshwater and Stickley's recommendation for greater use of the arts and humanities in EI education and curricula, educators have also used innovative and creative educational activities with students to enhance their understandings of their emotions and the importance of emotion work with patients. Warne and McAndrew (2008), for example, use painting as a self-reflective activity for nursing students, who are asked to reflect on their recent clinical work with specific patients. One learning activity involves asking the students to think about a patient they have cared for who has experienced some kind of loss, e.g. the loss of a relationship or a body part such as a limb, or the loss of self-esteem. Students then paint a picture representing the person and their loss and use colour to represent the person's mood. Once this is completed, students are then asked to paint themselves into the picture and to also use colour to reflect their own feelings while they were with the person. Warne and McAndrew (2008) found that such visual accounts of their experiences stimulated students and challenged their thinking about the patient, themselves, and their therapeutic work. Classroom discussion following the painting was used as a prompt for group learning and for making connections between theoretical concepts of the self and one's emotions, and the practice of therapeutic use of self and emotion work. Warne and McAndrew (2008) used these activities as opportunities for critical reflexive discussion of the student's self in relation to the patient and as a way to enhance students' self-insight. As may be evident to the reader, this potentially transformative teaching activity may also contribute to a transformatory learning experience for the educator.

Another creative activity useful for reflective practice and reflexivity is the use of narrative writing, or story exploration. Bolton (2006), for instance, has worked with health professionals and asked them write stories and poetry as part of reflections on their practice. The professionals are encouraged to write as if they were a patient or student who was impartially observing everything that happens, or to write for children, or as a child, about what they do. This method of enquiry uses a narrative approach within dialogical small groups and draws on the transformative power of expressive writing to develop practical wisdom from experience, to strengthen health professionals' ability to listen, and to increase their understandings of patient experiences. Such a process can also extend the practitioners' ability to demonstrate empathy.

Developing empathy

Empathy is widely cited as a key component of EI, and strengthening health and social care professionals' ability to demonstrate empathy is a common theme in the literature (Cadman and Brewer 2001, Freshwater and Stickley 2004, Grewal and Davidson 2008, Hurley 2008, Roberts 2010, Stratton *et al.* 2008). This is particularly in relation to health and social care professionals' ability to move from understanding the 'self' to understanding and supporting the 'other'. In trying to understand a situation from another person's perspective, being empathetic can be understood through the metaphor of 'putting yourself in someone else's shoes'. Empathy is the ability to understand another person from *his or her* perspective and expressed point of view (rather than one's own). Empathy involves observing, listening, understanding and attending to another and as such requires considerable use of communication skills (Usher, Foster and Luck 2009).

However, it is important to note that being technically proficient in interpersonal communication skills will not necessarily confer empathic ability on the communicator, but rather will provide a vehicle through which empathy may be developed. Horsfall, Stuhlmiller and Champ (2000) reinforce that empathy involves being able to put our own needs aside to be available to other people and to perceive their feelings and personal experience. In doing so, it enables us to interpersonally connect within a therapeutic relationship – empathy is considered one of the most crucial components of EI.

For health professionals, the relationship between empathy and compassion may also be critical. While empathy enables *understanding* of another's situation, it is the feeling of compassion that frequently underpins human *responses* to suffering and misfortune. Philosopher Martha Nussbaum (1996) identifies compassion as a basic human emotion, arguing that there is an element of self-interest in our compassionate responses to the suffering of others. In fact, she suggests that, given the inevitability of suffering in human societies and the social nature of human existence, the survival of our species does to a large extent depend on our compassionate responses to the pain of others. In a globalised world, however, where we are continually exposed to images and stories of suffering on a massive scale, people increasingly experience 'compassion fatigue', which some scholars argue can make it difficult for them to respond with compassion within their own personal lives (*see* Mestrovic 1997, for example). It is important, then, for health professionals to think critically about the nature of empathy and compassion, and the ways in which their own emotional experiences and responses might interact with those of their patients.

From this perspective, educational initiatives designed to strengthen health and social care professionals' abilities not only to *empathise with* but to *understand* their own compassionate responses to suffering are likely to go some way towards addressing the difficulties students experience when faced with the complexities and messiness of the lives of those they seek to help. In a study exploring medical students' personal experiences with patient-centredness, Bombeke and colleagues (2010) point to a number of barriers to students being able to maintain their focus on providing patient-centred care. In this study, medical students claimed that the lack of interest on the part of educators in the 'student-as-person' limited their professional development and their ability to deal with emotions and personal suffering. Students, mostly with limited exposure to life experiences, described being overwhelmed by suffering. One young student on a hospital placement explained: 'How are you yourself supposed to deal with all the misery you see … There's an awful lot of suffering hitting you straight in the face'. Suchman (2006) argues for an emphasis in healthcare on relationship-centred care, stating that this approach can also be extended to the education arena through the use of 'relationship-centred teaching'. He contends that this approach enables students to grapple with complexity and their own place/role within that complexity.

Given that many beginning health professional students have limited life experiences and that they can be 'overwhelmed by suffering' during their early clinical practicum, we have found that there are significant benefits to be gained by creatively engaging students in learning activities that have the potential to develop EI. This can be done in a 'safe' learning environment through activities that increase students' awareness and understanding of how individual people experience and make sense of their own suffering, and how healthcare professionals can, through developing empathy and understanding their own compassionate responses, engage in relationship-centred care without being overwhelmed by the suffering that confronts them. We have developed a learning activity for a large cohort of pre-registration nursing students that is designed to be used early in their education program to help strengthen their ability to demonstrate empathy and manage their own compassionate feelings.

Empathy learning activities

For this activity, students initially work in groups of three or four. As a group they are allocated a case study involving an imaginary person with a particular illness. The case study provides brief information about the person's illness and social situation. For a class of approximately 30 students there are two case studies available. This means that there may be several groups working on each case study. Students are required to explore the qualitative research literature on that illness experience, and then each group develops a script for an interview with the imaginary person in their case study, exploring their likely personal experience of a particular illness. The idea is for students to work together to think about how the illness might be experienced in the full context of that person's life, to develop an understanding of *how* it might feel and *what* it might mean to that person to be experiencing *that* illness at *that* point in *their* life.

Several groups work on each case study, and thus several imaginary interviews are developed from the one case study. Prior to a scheduled class, students are asked to read all the scripts that have been developed from their own case study. When the class meets, students will work together to discuss what they have found and why they have developed their interview in a particular way. The tutor works with each class to thematically analyse the information contained in all of the interviews based on the two case studies so that the whole class develops a beginning understanding of what is known about personal experiences of two particular illnesses. Two case studies about different cancer illness experiences, for example, might identify issues such as discrimination in the workplace, loss of friends, or discomfort because of changed physical appearance. These might be conceptualised as indicating stigmatisation of cancer illnesses. At the conclusion of the analysis session, five or six themes may have been developed that seem to encapsulate that illness experience.

Students are then asked to independently write an essay about the illness experience that was the focus of their case study in response to a question that challenges them to explore in depth issues of suffering such as emotionality, loss, isolation and/or uncertainty. Activities such as this have the potential to facilitate the development or strengthening of EI for each student, and the activity is positioned quite early in the course program so that students can benefit prior to experiencing too many confronting situations in real healthcare settings. The focus of this complex pyramid activity is on developing students' self-awareness, mindfulness and EI. The intention is to assist students to build their confidence about being involved in intimate health professional–patient relationships that may be emotionally complex and confronting. While engaged in this extended activity, students are also attending lectures, including at least one presented by people who have experienced serious illnesses, and reading texts that focus on complementary subject matter. Feedback from students indicates that by the time they have completed their essays, they are considerably more aware than they had been at the start of this subject about the issues faced by people with serious illnesses and about the inevitably emotional nature of their experiences.

There are, of course, many other learning activities that can contribute in similar ways.

Another very effective and commonly used strategy to facilitate learning about patient experiences and to develop EI is to bring students together with people who have themselves experienced serious physical and/or mental illnesses. This can be done with small and large groups and provides students with an opportunity to talk with people who have been consumers or 'patients' about their personal illness narratives and their experiences of interacting with health professionals. The view of this chapter's authors, in line with Clarke's (2010), is that these experiences are likely to be particularly productive for student development when they are shared with other students and with educators within a team-based, collaborative learning framework.

Of course, clinical placement initiatives are also extremely important, situated, educational experiences that offer relatively unexplored opportunities for developing and evaluating EI in pre-registration students. It is here, in the context of 'real' healthcare settings, that students can most effectively 'test' or 'try out' their own EI abilities. In this context, clinical supervisors and facilitators have very significant roles to play in supporting students to explore their EI abilities, particularly their self-awareness and use of self in therapeutic relationships.

Developing interpersonal relationships and communication skills

Self-awareness and the use of self are integral aspects of the interpersonal patient–practitioner relationship. The practitioner's ability to form caring and therapeutic relationships is considered the foundation of one's work, and thus the interpersonal relationship is considered a central component of EI (Roberts 2010, Hurley 2008). The ability to form effective interpersonal relationships calls upon both intrapersonal (self-awareness, empathy) and interpersonal (effective communication), intelligences, or EI (McQueen 2004). These enable the practitioner to manage his or her own and others' emotions – in other words, to do emotion work (Hurley 2008, McQueen 2004). This ability to be 'emotionally resonant' or 'affectively attuned' to patients is a necessary part of effective patient–practitioner relationships (Roberts 2010).

The concept of 'emotion work' has been central to the work of Arlie Hochschild, who sought to understand what it is that people actually 'think or do' about the feelings they have. She stated that individuals have the capacity to 'work' on an uncomfortable or 'inappropriate' feeling to attempt to produce an emotional state that is more 'acceptable', either to the individual or within a particular context. She argued that each community, society or social group has its own socially constructed 'feeling rules', which identify 'guidelines for the assessment of fits and misfits between feeling and situation' (1979, p. 566). Famously, Hochschild went on to claim that this capacity for responding to feeling rules to produce emotions that are acceptable within given social situations has been commercialised by organisations that require employees to continually present a 'positive' persona within the workplace.

Hochschild's thesis has been the subject of much debate (for example, *see* Barbalet 1998); nevertheless it has been very influential beyond its original application within the airline industry. The concepts of emotion work and emotional labour have been widely applied within health and social care, particularly nursing (for example, *see* Dingwall and Allen 2001, Bolton 2001), and have been linked to the broader concept of EI. While they are separate constructs, emotional labour (EL) relies upon EI in that it involves the use of intra- and interpersonal intelligences (McQueen 2004).

The theory of EL has been extended by other researchers in health and social care. Theodosius (2008) for instance, developed a three-factor framework of EL in nursing which can be applied to the use of communication skills. The framework includes: **collegial EL**, the relationships and communication health and social care professionals have with each other; **instrumental EL**, the use of communication skills to facilitate a clinical intervention or procedure, e.g. giving an injection; and **therapeutic EL**, the use of communication skills to establish or maintain a therapeutic relationship with a patient in order to promote their psychological or emotional well-being.

The interpersonal patient–practitioner relationship is dependent on a number of factors, including the practitioner's self-awareness, self-management, and ability to show empathy. Communication microskills form a part of the skill set practitioners need to form and maintain an effective patient–practitioner relationship. Education in interpersonal communication is a common aspect of health and social care education, and there are numerous books outlining various models for communication and activities for building students' capacity to gain rapport with patients, to listen effectively, and to facilitate emotional expression with their patients. It is not our intention to replicate these here. Instead we outline particular activities we have developed and found useful in building students' communication and interpersonal skills.

Interpersonal and communication skills learning activities

Microskills, i.e. non-verbal and verbal skills used in interpersonal communication, are commonly taught in health and social care programs. One approach in teaching these skills that we have found effective is based on a model outlined by Geldard and Geldard (2005). Students work in groups of three (the triad model) – with one as patient, one as health and social care practitioner, and one as observer. The students are given handouts to record observations for each of six microskills (joining and listening; reflection of content; reflection of feelings; reflection of both content and feelings; use of questions; and summarising). Students will have already received lectures and readings on communication and these microskills prior to their skills practice. Educators role-play the skills prior to students practising them.

Students then take turns in role-playing a real-life, everyday problem or situation they have experienced that they are comfortable sharing with others, e.g. anxiety about exams, or perhaps frustration with traffic delays. This assists with building more authentic responses from the 'patient' and the 'practitioner'. Students share the roles and practise one microskill at a time, rotating through each role and skill so they all perform as the practitioner for at least two of the skills. They then practice drawing all the skills together in one interaction. We have found using this model with the observer role to be effective, because the verbal and written feedback students receive from each other provides a structured form of peer feedback that is focused and constructive.

Role-playing is a teaching tool commonly used to simulate real-life experiences for students so they can experiment in a safe setting with professional practitioner responses. In terms of interpersonal skills and communication training, educators can demonstrate appropriate responses to particular situations, with educators, students, or in some cases, actors, playing the role of a patient or family member. This can be a very effective use of valuable classroom time, as relatively large groups of students can observe, and then practice, particular communication and interpersonal skills. Using an incremental learning approach in a practice session which follows from the previous session on microskills, we have used paid actors to portray patients or family members with anxiety, agitation and/or distress. The focus is on interacting with a person in distress and managing his and the other person's emotional responses. Students are grouped into small groups of four or five and given a brief outline of the situation. Drawing on their microskills knowledge, they discuss how they would approach the person (actor) and what questions they might need to ask. Each group then interacts with the actor, with one student starting off the interaction and subsequent students taking over and continuing the conversation. Large group discussion, with the actor sharing his responses to the varying approaches and students observing how others approach the same situation, has been very effective for student learning. At the end of the class, the facilitator or a student may conduct an entire interaction to show how the microskills can be effectively applied to build rapport and to manage the person's emotional distress.

CONCLUSION

This chapter has outlined a range of theories and approaches for educating adult learners in the health and social care professions and helping develop their EI knowledge and abilities. While the theoretical underpinnings of these approaches have been discussed, the focus has been on sharing the authors' personal approaches and others' interactive and/or innovative EI-enhancing activities. The aim has been to stimulate educators and learners' own creativity and to provide a toolkit of activities useful for developing EI programs in a range of contexts and health and social care practitioner groups.

FURTHER LEARNING ACTIVITIES AND RESOURCES

Table 10.4 provides a summary of activities for identifying, using, understanding and managing emotions. These are based on Mayer and Salovey's four-factor model of EI (*see* Chapter 1, Introducing emotional intelligence).

Creative resources for emotional intelligence education
Film
Look Both Ways (2005) – This Australian film can facilitate discussion about emotions that can arise with serious, life-threatening diagnoses, and the ways in which such events are inevitably experienced within complicated human lives involving many different kinds of relationships.

The Diving Bell and the Butterfly (2007) – This film is based on the real-life story of *Elle France* editor Jean-Dominique Bauby, who suffered a stroke that left him paralysed except for the use of one eye. The film can stimulate discussion about

TABLE 10.4 Activities for identifying, using, understanding and managing emotion

Identifying emotions
- The ability to identify emotions can be strengthened through active observation of facial expressions and noting their congruence/lack of congruence with the person's spoken words and tone of voice, e.g. through role-playing and validation of observations with the person (Caruso and Wolfe 2001, in: Vitello-Cicciu 2002).
- Clinical placements (particularly those where patients are seriously or critically ill) can facilitate students' ability to identify emotions in others. Include patient care debriefings to discuss patient/family emotional reactions and student responses.
- Use a mood journal to facilitate self-reflection (during semester and/or clinical placement), e.g. What am I feeling now? What cues (verbal or non-verbal) am I sending to others?

Using emotions in thought
- In situations where people are distressed, learn how to activate listening skills to remain in the present, i.e. be empathic, then reflect and debrief on the resulting situation in order to learn from it, e.g. in clinical supervision.

Understanding and analysing emotions
- Learn about the role emotional plays in constructing meaning in relationships, and about the transition of emotions from one state to another, e.g. annoyance or irritation developing into rage.
- Learn about the range and types of emotions, what causes them, and how emotions function, e.g. understanding that anger can be the result of fear, or the perception of being wronged or experiencing an injustice.
- Role-play emotional situations and analyse them afterward, e.g. the communication activity we have used with students in the previous chapter activities
- Stories or narratives of clinical situations depicting challenging emotions can be used to enhance learners' ability to recognise, interpret and respond to interpersonal situations.
- Mentors and/or coaches can provide support and role modelling in handling challenging situations in the workplace.

Managing emotions
- The ability to generate emotions to solve problems or calm oneself before an emotional event, i.e. emotional labour, can be developed through relaxation training, breathing techniques and visualisation exercises.

(Adapted from Vitello-Cicciu 2002)

emotions and the roles of healthcare professionals in supporting people in very difficult social and health-related circumstances.

Literature

Tiger's Eye – a Memoir (2001) – Inga Clendinnen's work is a fascinating reflection by the author on her experience with acute liver disease. The story interweaves memories from Inga's life with her emotional responses to her illness and the circumstances that prompted those responses. This book can facilitate discussion of how complex illness experiences can be; it also addresses relationships with healthcare professionals and interactions with other patients.

Art and music

Vincent Van Gogh's series of self portraits and work *The Starry Night* and Don McLean's song *Vincent* can be used in teaching about mental illness (particularly psychosis) and/or suicidality. The authors of this chapter have used the combination of *The Starry Night* and *Vincent* as an evocative introduction to illustrating Van Gogh's decline in mental health over time, coupled with his life story. Van Gogh's story illustrates the impact of stigma and the suffering that can occur for individuals and their families. The combination of artwork, music and story are a powerful way to evoke empathy, encourage reflective discussion on mental illness, and facilitate development of effective strategies that can be used to counter these impacts.

REFERENCES

Bandura A. *Social Learning Theory.* New York: General Learning Press; 1977.

Barbalet J. *Emotion, Social Theory and Social Structure: a macrosociological approach.* Cambridge: Cambridge University Press; 1998.

Bellack JP. Emotional intelligence: a missing ingredient? *J Nurs Educ.* 1999; **38**(1): 3–4.

Bleakley A. Blunting Occam's razor: aligning medical education with studies of complexity. *J Eval Clin Pract.* 2010; **16**(4): 849–55.

Bolton G. Narrative writing: reflective enquiry into professional practice. *Educational Action Research.* 2006; **14**(2): 203–18.

Bolton S. Changing faces: nurses as emotional jugglers. *Sociology of Health & Illness.* 2001; **23**(1): 85–100.

Bombecke K, Symons L, Debaene L, *et al.* Help, I'm losing patient-centredness! Experiences of medical students and their teachers. *Med Educ.* 2010; **44**(7): 662–73.

Cadman C, Brewer J. Emotional intelligence: a vital prerequisite for recruitment in nursing. *J Nurs Manag.* 2001: **9**(6); 321–4.

Cherniss C. *Emotional Intelligence: what it is and why it matters.* Paper presented at: the annual meeting of the Society for Industrial and Organizational Psychology; 15 April 2000; New Orleans, LA. Available at: www.eiconsortium.org/reports/what_is_emotional_intelligence.html (accessed 20 February 2008).

Cherniss C, Goleman D, Emmerling R, *et al.* 1998 *Guidelines for Best Practice.* Available at: www.eiconsortium.org/reports/guidelines.html (accessed 18 July 2011).

Clarke N. Emotional intelligence training: a case of caveat emptor. *Human Resource Development Review.* 2006; **5**(4): 422–41.

Clarke N. Developing emotional intelligence abilities through team-based learning. *Human Resource Development Quarterly.* 2010; **21**(2): 119–38.

Clouder L, Sellars J. Reflective practice and clinical supervision: an interprofessional perspective. *J Adv Nurs.* 2004; **46**(3): 262–9.

Dingwall R, Allen D. The implications of healthcare reforms for the profession of nursing. *Nurs Inq.* 2001; **8**: 64–74.

Foster K, McAllister M, O'Brien L. Extending the boundaries: autoethnography as an emergent method in mental health nursing research. *Int J Ment Health Nurs.* 2006; **15**(1): 44–53.

Foster K, Usher K, Gadai S, *et al.* There is no health without mental health: implementing the first mental health nursing program in Fiji. *Contemp Nurse.* 2009; **32**(1–2): 179–86.

Freshwater D, Stickley TJ. The heart of the art: emotional intelligence in nurse education. *Nurs Inq.* 2004; **11**(2): 91–8.

Gallop R, O'Brien L. Re-establishing psychodynamic theory as foundational knowledge for psychiatric/mental health nursing. *Issues Ment Health Nurs.* 2003; **24**(2): 213–27.

Geldard D, Geldard K. *Basic Personal Counselling: a training manual for counsellors.* 5th ed. Frenchs Forest: Pearson Education; 2005.

Grewal D, Davidson HA. Emotional intelligence and graduate medical education. *JAMA.* 2008; **300**(10): 1200–2.

Harrison PA, Fopma-Loy JL. Reflective journal prompts: a vehicle for stimulating emotional competence in nursing. *J Nurs Educ* [online advanced release]. 2010; **49**(11): 644–52.

Hochschild A. Emotion work, feeling rules, and social structure. *American Journal of Sociology.* 1979; **85**(3): 551–75.

Horsfall J, Stuhlmiller C, Champ S. *Interpersonal Nursing for Mental Health.* Sydney: MacLennan & Petty; 2000.

Hurley J. The necessity, barriers and ways forward to meet user-based needs for emotionally intelligent nurses. *J Psychiatr Ment Health Nurs.* 2008; **15**(5): 379–85.

Jackson D, O'Brien L. The effective nurse. In: Elder R, Evans K, Nizette D, editors. *Psychiatric and Mental Health Nursing.* 2nd ed. Sydney: Elsevier; 2009. pp. 2–11.

Knowles M. *Andragogy in Action: applying modern principles of adult learning.* San Francisco, CA: Jossey-Bass; 1984.

Levett-Jones TL. Self-directed learning: implications and limitations for undergraduate nursing education. *Nurse Educ Today.* 2005; **25**(5): 363–8.

Luft H. *Of Human Interaction.* Palo Alto, CA: Mayfield; 1969.

Mayer J, Salovey P. What is emotional intelligence? In: Salovey P, Sluyter D, editors. *Emotional Development and Emotional Intelligence: implications for educators.* New York, NY: Basic Books; 1997. pp. 3–31.

McAllister M. Transformative teaching in nursing education: preparing for the possible. *Collegian.* 2005; **12**(1): 13–18.

McQueen ACH. Emotional intelligence in nursing work. *J Adv Nurs.* 2004; **47**(1): 101–8.

McWilliam E, Hatcher C. Emotional literacy as a pedagogical product. *Continuum: Journal of Media & Cultural Studies.* 2004; **18**(2): 179–89.

Mennin S. Complexity and health professions education. *J Eval Clin Pract.* 2010; **16**(4): 835–7.

Mestrovic S. *Postemotional Society.* London: Sage; 1997.

Mezirow J. Transformative learning: theory to practice. In: Cranton P, editor. *Transformative Learning in Action: insights from practice. New Directions for Adult and Continuing Education no. 74.* San Francisco, CA: Jossey-Bass; 1997. pp. 5–12.

Mezirow J. *Learning as transformation: critical perspectives on a theory in progress.* San Francisco, CA: Jossey-Bass; 2000.

Nussbaum M. Compassion: the basic social emotion. *Social Philosophy & Policy.* 1996; **13**(1): 27–38.

Roberts M. Emotional intelligence, empathy and the educative power of poetry: a Deleuzo-Guattarian perspective. *J Psychiatr Ment Health Nurs.* 2010; **17**(3): 236–41.

Stratton TD, Saunders JA, Elam CL. Changes in medical students' emotional intelligence: an exploratory study. *Teach Learn Med.* 2008; **20**(3): 279–84.

Suchman A. A new theoretical foundation for relationship centred care: complex responsive processes of relating. *J Gen Intern Med.* 2006; **21**(Suppl. 1): S40–4.

Theodosius C. *Emotional Labour in Healthcare: the unmanaged heart of nursing.* London: Routledge; 2008.

Usher K, Foster K, Luck L. The patient as person. In: Elder R, Evans K, Nizette D, op. cit. pp. 408–28.

Usher K, Foster K, Stewart L. Reflective practice for the graduate nurse. In: Chang E, Daly J, editors. *Transitions in Nursing: preparing for professional practice.* Sydney: Elsevier; 2008. pp. 275–89.

Vitello-Cicciu JM. Exploring emotional intelligence: implications for nursing leaders. *J Nurs Adm.* 2002; **32**(4): 203–10.

Warne T, McAndrew S. Painting the landscape of emotionality: colouring in the emotional gaps between theory and practice of mental health nursing. *Int J Ment Health Nurs.* 2008; **17**(2): 108–15.

Wouters C. The sociology of emotions and flight attendants: Hochschild's managed heart. *Theory, Culture & Society.* 1989; **6**(1): 95–123.

CHAPTER 11

Some final thoughts on emotional intelligence

John Hurley and Paul Linsley

Throughout this book, the chapter authors, practitioners and educators from across a spectrum of international settings and professional disciplines have spoken about and applied EI to the daily roles of health and social care practice. As the reader of this text, you have been invited to reflect upon yourself as both a person and a professional in terms of your EI capabilities, and how you might use these capabilities when around others in your workplace settings. Hopefully, such reflections have been a journey of growth for you.

EI has also been forwarded as a foundational capability upon which your capacity to effectively assist and develop others and your own professional progression is built around. Through breaking down the term EI into its individual capability components it is hoped that you have been able to identify and think about how you might use these in your roles as a nurse, social worker, occupational therapist, or doctor of medicine. Importantly, EI has also been applied to how you can potentially be a more effective leader, as well as a better follower when this is required. The health and social care workplace has been offered as being at times a challenging one, often themed with imbalances of power and uncertainty. The identification of EI as a partial mitigation of such power imbalances offers a potentially new way to respond to these workplace challenges.

Ultimately, however, this text has sought to inspire you to reflect upon how you can provide better care to those in need of it through the use of EI capabilities. As we highlighted at the very beginning of this text, modern-day health and social care is pressured through decreasing contact time between the givers and recipients of care. Additionally, the increasing sophistication of treatments necessitates practitioners to prioritise the learning of how to be skilled in applying these treatments.

Within this pressured mix the recipients of care still need advanced interpersonal relating, and all the benefits that come directly and indirectly from that relating. Consequently, practitioners must be skilled not only in applying sophisticated treatments, but also in the art and science of effective 'human-to-human' relating. On the most basic of levels, recipients of care need sophisticated intervention delivered with advanced interpersonal skills to reach their maximum level of wellness. One without the other cannot achieve this end.

EMOTIONAL INTELLIGENCE AND EDUCATION

Hopefully by reading this book you will have reached the conclusion that your EI capabilities can be improved by firstly being aware of what they are, and then by consciously working on them. With full cognisance of the pressures on education and training agendas there arguably remains a need to give greater emphasis toward creating opportunities for developing EI capabilities. While they are recognisable within many of the educational and professional standards for health and social care across international perspectives, EI capabilities are at times *not* obvious within the teaching and learning programmes for health and social care professionals.

While some argument can be forwarded that EI capabilities are discernable within curricula, they are often buried within other topics or are implicit within the content, as distinct from being explicit within the learning outcomes and assessments of practitioner competence. Post qualifying education, training and continuing professional development can also lack overt recognition and priority toward both the interpersonal and intrapersonal capability development that is synonymous with EI.

This development of EI capabilities was shown through the work of Boyatzis (2002) and Cherniss *et al.* (1998) to be a change that must be self-driven toward what a person is inspired to become. Consequently, EI capabilities sought through health and social care policy educational strategies alone cannot be successfully implemented without practitioners being inspired to choose to adopt them. Building such inspiration may require health and social care stakeholders engaging in discourses that pay greater overt recognition toward such capabilities within both academic and workplace-based education and training, and the leadership to drive the agenda forward. Reinforcing the need for all categories of professionals to generate co-constructions toward successful EI enhancement is also required to generate workplace cultures that are safe for experimentation with the new behaviours emergent from such interpersonal and intrapersonal development (Boyatzis 2002, Cherniss *et al.* 1998).

Commencing such education and training under the framework of learning communities and through heutagogic learning approaches appears to be one potentially useful way forward. Heutagogy, or a self-determined approach to learning, acknowledges that people learn through random response to unpredictable needs, frequently when faced with the limits of their current knowledge or capabilities, reflective of the practice-based lifeworld (Hase and Kenyon 1999). Learning communities or communities of practice place a powerful emphasis on learning as a socially underpinned and practise-based exercise that highlight learning as being inherent within human nature (Wenger 1996). Pivotally, learning communities seek and acknowledge that learning develops and hence changes who the learner is, accurately reflecting important EI considerations and incorporating identity as being central to learning. Additionally, the workplace emphasis also reflects the learning preferences of many practitioners.

THE CHALLENGES FOR EMOTIONAL INTELLIGENCE IN HEALTH AND SOCIAL CARE

While the imperative to maximise the integration of EI into education and training for health and social care roles may appear to be blatantly obvious, there is also the need for caution. Akerjordet and Severinsson (2010) provide an excellent overview of the state of EI science and highlight many areas where the apparently blatantly obvious does in fact require careful consideration.

Nowhere within the variable constructs of EI are there explicit ethical boundaries to guide behaviours. One may simply use EI to achieve an end which is beneficial only to themselves, or for purposes that lay outside developing and/or caring for others. One may have EI capabilities but choose not to enact or implement them, despite knowing that this results in diminished professional functioning. One may also simply 'fake' EI behaviours on a day-to-day basis, sound in the knowledge that most EI tests are cumbersome and unlikely to be administered within a professional development review. Even if such a review were undertaken, the ethics of the organisation are equally unregulated by EI. Employers can simply determine which workplace employee behaviours are emotionally appropriate, and which are not. Given that developing EI capability is partially a personal commitment, one deeply connected to a sense of self and personal identity, such intrusions can be forwarded as being a potentially dangerous power for employers to have.

EI at its most fundamental level has been identified as the capacity to combine cognition and emotions toward reaching a desired outcome (Mayer and Salovey 1997). While the authors of this chapter and the other contributors to this book have focused on an 'applied' perspective of EI, one of its greatest challenges lies in establishing more rigorous empirical measures. There is a widening recognition that this capacity to utilise emotions and cognition is indeed intelligence, and there is also a growing consensus toward the capabilities and/or traits that make up this thing we are calling EI. However, the study of EI is a relatively new phenomenon, and dispute remains as to what precisely should be included under its umbrella term.

EI is hence clearly not a construct that solves all problems, nor is it a capability that is inherently and inevitably 'good' or 'nice'. EI, within the confines of its existing models, has no authority to make recommendations toward which emotions are positive or negative, which behaviours are acceptable or unacceptable or whether a professional is eligible for entry into a profession or for professional advancement. EI, like all other capabilities and intelligences, must be applied to the contexts in which it dwells. In other words, EI needs to be embedded within existing ethical and moral frameworks that guide and inform the behaviours of health and social care professionals. EI must also be a part of rather than be the sole determinate of performance, as the science of EI remains too embryonic for such absolute empirical application of it. We certainly echo the suggestions of Akerjordet and Severinsson (2010) in calling for advancing the quantitative research of EI by moving outwards from existing empirical studies and models, whilst simultaneously contextualising what we do know about EI to practice and educational settings.

CONCLUSION

Despite the psychometric disputes, there is little doubt that the recipients of care strongly desire and profoundly appreciate EI capabilities from their caregivers. Your task, as an educator, student or qualified professional, lies more with the application of EI to the work that you undertake. Be inspired to communicate your empathy, be diligent in honestly and regularly assessing yourself, and lead yourself and others in a manner which resonates with the stated values and ethics of your profession; by doing so, everyone benefits.

REFERENCES

Akerjordet K, Severinsson E. The state of the science of emotional intelligence related to nursing leadership: an integrative review. *J Nurs Manag.* 2010; **18**(4): 363–82.

Boyatzis R. Unleashing the power of self-directed learning. In: Sims R, editor. *Changing the Way We Manage Change: the consultants speak.* New York: Quorum Books; 2002. pp. 13–32. Available at: www.eiconsortium.org/reprints/self-directed_learning.html (accessed 18 July 2011).

Cherniss C, Goleman D, Emmerling R, *et al. Guidelines for Best Practice.* Available at: www.eiconsortium.org/reports/guidelines.html (accessed 18 July 2011).

Hase S, Kenyon C. From andragogy to heutagogy [unpublished paper]. Available at: http://ultibase.rmit.edu.au/Articles/dec00/hase1.pdf (accessed 18 July 2011).

Mayer J, Salovey P. What is emotional intelligence? In: Salovey P, Sluyter D, editors. *Emotional Development and Emotional Intelligence: implications for educators.* New York, NY: Basic Books; 1997. pp. 3–31.

Wenger E. Communities of practice: the social fabric of the learning organisation. *Healthc Forum J.* 1996; **39**(4): 20–6.

Index